Assessment Scales in Child and Adolescent Psychiatry

Assessment Scales in Child and Adolescent Psychiatry

Frank C Verhulst, MD, PhD
Professor and Director
Department of Child and Adolescent Psychiatry
Erasmus MC
Sophia Children's Hospital
Rotterdam
The Netherlands

Jan van der Ende, MS
Psychologist
Department of Child and Adolescent Psychiatry
Erasmus MC
Sophia Children's Hospital
Rotterdam
The Netherlands

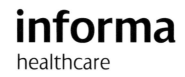

© 2006 Informa UK Ltd

First published in the United Kingdom in 2006 by Informa UK Ltd, 4 Park Square, Milton Park,
Abingdon, Oxon OX14 4RN
Informa Healthcare is a trading division of Informa UK Ltd,
Registered Office: 37/41 Mortimer Street, London W1T 3JH. Registered in England and Wales
Number 1072954.

Tel: +44 (0)20 7017 6000
Fax: +44 (0)20 7017 6699
Email: info.medicine@tandf.co.uk
Website: www.tandf.co.uk/medicine

A CIP record for this book is available from the British Library.
Library of Congress Cataloging-in-Publication Data

Data available on application

ISBN10 1 84184 534 5
ISBN13 978 1 84184 534 0

Distributed in North and South America by
Taylor & Francis
6000 Broken Sound Parkway, NW, (Suite 300)
Boca Raton, FL 33487, USA

Within Continental USA
Tel: 800 272 7737; Fax: 800 374 3401
Outside Continental USA
Tel: 561 994 0555; Fax: 561 361 6018
Email: orders@crcpress.com

Distributed in the rest of the world by
Thomson Publishing Services
Cheriton House
North Way
Andover, Hampshire SP10 5BE, UK
Tel: +44 (0)1264 332424
Email: tps.tandfsalesorder@thomson.com

Composition by Scribe Design Ltd, Ashford, Kent, UK
Printed and bound in Italy by Printer Trento S.r.l.

Contents

Preface

The assessment and diagnosis of child and adolescent psychopathology has been the main focus of our research over the last twenty years. When the publisher approached us to write a book containing a comprehensive collection of rating scales for assessing psychopathology in children and adolescents, we did not hesitate to do so, because such an enterprise fitted nicely into our own wish to have access to a reference source on existing rating scales for our own and our colleagues' research and clinical practice.

The complexity of factors involved in the assessment and diagnosis of child and adolescent psychopathology makes this an especially intriguing field. The need for multiple informants (e.g. parents, teachers, and the children themselves), the role of age and developmental change, and the quantitative rather than qualitative nature of child psychopathology are major factors that need to be taken into account when dealing with the measurement of child and adolescent emotional and behavioral problems. Since the recognition that assessment procedures need to be standardized, reliable and valid, and since the introduction of instruments that fitted these criteria, clinical work and research have benefited greatly from reproducible and quantifiable information that was obtained with these procedures.

There are different approaches to the assessment of child psychopathology, including clinical interviews, psychological tests, and rating scales. This book is on rating scales. Rating scales have the advantage that they can be used in a variety of settings in a cost-effective way. Because rating scales can be easily applied to large numbers of subjects, often rating scales have norms that can be used to compare an individual child to same-aged peers. We have attempted to list the majority of rating scales that have been published. The only criterion for inclusion was the availability of enough psychometric properties of a scale to enable the reader to make a judgment. We have approached authors and/or publishers to provide us with the most up to date versions and documentation of the scales. For each scale we have asked permission to reproduce the scale, either in full form, or as sample items. We have attempted to give information about each scale as accurately as possible in an objective and structured way. We had to rely either on commercially available materials (such as manuals) or on published reports in peer-reviewed journals. We are grateful to many authors and publishers who were supportive and helped us by providing us with materials and suggestions.

We have not attempted to give recommendations on the use of scales, since different scales may be appropriate for different purposes. In the introduction we have given a number of guidelines the reader might find useful for choosing a certain scale. We recommend that the original publication on scales is consulted before a scale can be used.

Most rating scales were designed in the English language, and for the majority of scales norms are based on US or UK populations. In our rapidly changing society in which many children from various cultural backgrounds live together in one geographical area and with the increasing use of rating scales in countries where the native language in non-English, it is helpful to know if a rating scale is available in different languages and whether local norms are available. For some scales this information is available, but for the majority of scales this is not the case. Because systematic information on translations and local norms was lacking for the majority of scales, we have omitted this information in this edition. Hopefully it will be possible to include this important information in a next edition.

We wish to thank the publisher for taking the initiative to publish this book and Abigail Griffin, Kelly Cornish and Peter Stevenson for supporting us to accomplish this in due time.

Frank C Verhulst
Jan van der Ende

Chapter 1

Introduction

There is a wealth of rating scales for use in assessing child and adolescent psychopathology in both clinical and research settings. The choice of a rating scale will depend upon the purpose for which it will be used, and on its psychometric properties. Therefore, it is useful to have a comprehensive overview of existing rating scales to assess child and adolescent psychopathology, and to apply criteria for judging which scale best suits a particular purpose. This book presents a comprehensive collection of existing scales to assess child and adolescent psychopathology. Both generic instruments covering a wide range of psychopathology as well as disorder-specific scales are presented. There will be no focus upon the measurement of other concepts that may be relevant to the study of child and adolescent functioning, including neurocognitive functioning, temperament, personality, self-esteem, coping, or family functioning.

In this introduction, a number of principles underlying the construction and use of rating scales for the assessment of child/adolescent psychopathology will be presented. These principles are important for the evaluation of scales that may be relevant for certain purposes.

Issues specific to the assessment of child and adolescent psychopathology

Although relevant to the assessment and diagnosis of child/adolescent problem behavior in general, a number of issues are pertinent to the principles underlying the construction and use of rating scales. These issues are: (i) the age-relatedness of problem behavior; (ii) the informant and situational specificity of ratings; and (iii) the quantitative nature of many child/adolescent problem behaviors.

Age-relatedness

Many problem behaviors, such as temper tantrums or school refusal, may be regarded as normal at a young age, whereas these behaviors will be labeled as abnormal at older ages. To determine whether a child's behavior is deviant, we have to take account of the child's

developmental level. This is especially relevant for procedures, which are followed by decisions about individuals, including the decision to refer a particular child or adolescent for more specialized services, to begin a certain intervention, or to do a more extensive diagnostic assessment.

For children and adolescents who are within the normal range with respect to cognitive and physical development, comparisons with normative samples of children of the same age (and sex as well) provide guidelines for evaluating problems. If the ages of children in a sample differ significantly from the ages of children from whom standard ratings were obtained, it is not possible to make valid comparisons.

Some rating scales employ the same version for different age groups. This has the advantage that scores obtained for children at a certain age can be compared with scores obtained for the same children at a later age. In order to take into account the developmental aspect of behavior, it is important to use different norms for different ages. The relative level of problems of individuals from one age group can then be compared with those of individuals from another age group.

There are also rating scales that use different versions for different age groups, usually for preschool age, school age, and adolescence. Rating scales that use different versions for different age groups have the advantage that behaviors that are relevant for a certain age group but not for another are only included in the version for the relevant age group. For example, alcohol and drug use, truancy, or vandalism is relevant for the assessment of adolescents but not for preschool children. A disadvantage of the use of different versions for different age groups is that with the crossing from one age group to the other, we may lose continuity of item and scale scores. This is especially problematic for longitudinal research where complete continuity of item and scale scores is important.

Informant and situational specificity

When using rating scales, it is important to obtain information from different sources. Informants such as parents and teachers, who see children in different situations (home, classroom, playground) are needed to obtain a comprehensive picture of the child's functioning.

Parents are usually familiar with their child's functioning in many situations and across time. Teachers have the opportunity to compare a child's functioning with that of large groups of peers. Teacher reports may reveal difficulties in academic and social skills that may not be evident to parents. Adolescents may sometimes take the teacher into confidence and reveal significant problems to the teacher that the parents are unaware of. In addition to adults as informants, adolescents' self-reports are indispensable, especially on their own affective and other internalizing problems.

However, different informants having different relations to the child and seeing the child under different conditions, often vary in their response to the child's behavior. In a meta-analysis, Achenbach, McConaughy and Howell (1987) computed the average correlation between different informants' ratings of problem behaviors in a large number of published samples. The mean correlation between pairs of adult informants who played different roles with respect to the children was 0.28. The mean correlation between self-reports and reports by parents, teachers, and mental health workers was even lower (0.22). In contrast, the mean correlation between pairs of similar informants (e.g. father and mother; teacher and teacher aide) was 0.60.

The informants' differing standards for judging the child's functioning, as well as their specific impacts on the child and the situational specificity of the child's behavior, all are reflected in cross-informant variation. Children's behavior is often much more variable than that of adults, and children are more susceptible to environmental influences.

Instead of viewing low agreement between different informants as a nuisance, or systematically discarding one source of information, it is important to regard each informant as a potentially valid source of information. Each informant has its own, unique and potentially valid contribution to the formation of an overall picture of the child's functioning (Verhulst et al. 1994, 1997). Even disagreement among informants can be valuable (Jensen et al. 1999). For example, a child who used to be cheerful at school but who, quite suddenly, appears unhappy and withdrawn according to the teacher, but whose parents do not report any significant problem in the child's functioning at home, may be subjected to negative environmental influences in the home situation. Another example of the potential value of information from different sources is the finding that children who are hyperactive at home *and* at school have a poorer prognosis than children who are hyperactive at home *or* at school (Schachar, Rutter and Smith 1981).

Most rating scales have parallel versions for parents and teachers. Some scales have versions for adolescents' self-

reports, although for some rating scales the self-report version is not parallel to the parent and teacher versions and may tap other domains such as personality.

The advantage of rating scales with parallel parent, teacher and self-report versions is that the scores across the different informants can be compared. By comparing the level of agreement between different informants' reports on an individual child's problems with the level of agreement between similar informants typically found for large reference samples, it is possible to decide whether the reports by a particular pair of informants agree better, worse, or about the same as typically found between these two types of informants.

The dimensional nature of child/adolescent problem behaviors

The construction of rating scales is usually based on psychometric principles. The basic premise is that most problem behaviors in children and adolescents can best be regarded as quantitative variations rather than either present or absent categories. In order to identify quantitative gradations in behavioral and emotional problems, multiple items, usually close-ended questions, are scored by the respondent. This is done following standardized procedures. In this way, errors arising from procedural variation are minimized.

To provide quantitative scores for different aspects of functioning, the items of rating scales are usually aggregated into scales. For instance, scores for each item of a rating scale with a large pool of items can be summarized into scale scores such as 'hyperactivity', 'anxiety', or 'oppositional'.

This quantitative approach makes it possible to assess the degree to which an individual child's or adolescent's problems deviates from that of same-sex age-mates in normative samples. Most assessment procedures employing rating scales use norms; however, the quality of the normative samples can vary considerably. Some use large representative samples from the general population, others use samples of convenience.

The advantage of using quantitative scores is that they contain more statistical information than categories. Due to their idiosyncratic nature, individual items are assumed to produce responses that are subject to error. By focussing on the consistency of answers across many items, and by disregarding the responses to individual questions, measurement error is reduced (Streiner and Norman 1998). Therefore the reliability of rating scales, which contain many items for sampling each aspect of functioning in a quantitative way, is often higher than that for categories that are scored as either present or absent.

The use of quantitative scores does not preclude the use of categories by employing cut-off points for distinguishing between cases and non-cases. However, the dividing line to define whether or not something is a case is not clear and rather arbitrary, although there are procedures to determine cut-off points that serve certain purposes best.

Overview of rating scales

The literature has been searched for psychometrically sound rating scales for the assessment of child/adolescent psychopathology. Questionnaires that were designed for very limited purposes, such as for particular research purposes only, have not been included. The authors and/or publishers were then contacted and information was requested on the format, administration, scoring and interpretation of the specific questionnaires as well as for permission to reproduce the scales either in whole or as sample items.

Focus has been concentrated on the application of criteria for evaluating the characteristics of rating scales, because they may aid in judging the usefulness of a particular instrument for certain purposes.

The quality of an instrument can be judged by a number of characteristics, including: applicability, acceptability, practicality, reliability, validity, and sensitivity to change.

In the main text an overview has been given of the rating scales that were selected. The aim was to provide a comprehensive description of the characteristics of each instrument. Information was extracted as much as possible from information obtained from the authors/publishers such as manuals, information sheets, scoring forms, as well as from published literature in peer-reviewed journals concerning these questionnaires.

Characteristics of rating scales

Item content

The content of the items of an instrument is of course chosen on the basis of what the instrument is intended to measure. For generic instruments this is a broad range of psychopathology, whereas for disorder specific instruments this will be only one domain such as anxiety, hyperactivity, depression or pervasive developmental disorder. A number of sources can serve as the basis for the selection of items, including clinical observations, expert opinions on item content, or key informants such as parents, teachers and children for whom the instruments are designed. Most rating scales use a mix of these sources to select the items. Another approach is the use of consensus among experts about the combination of

criteria for certain disorders as described in the literature or in classification systems such as the *Diagnostic and Statistical Manual of Mental Disorders* (DSM; American Psychiatric Association 1994). Authors of scales using this approach took the diagnostic criteria for DSM-IV categories that are relevant for children and adolescents as the item source for their instruments.

For scales that have been developed over many years through successive revisions, empirical information obtained from earlier versions (for instance on content coverage or on the discriminative validity of specific items) are incorporated into the newer versions. Examples are *The Achenbach System of Empirically Based Assessment* (ASEBA; Achenbach and Rescorla 1999) and the *Conners' Rating Scales-Revised* (CRS-R; Conners 1997). In the revision of the Conners' Rating Scales, Conners included items that were modelled on the DSM-IV criteria.

Item response scaling

Most rating scales have items that can be scored on a 3-point scale (0, 1 and 2), whereas some use 4-point scaling (0, 1, 2, and 3), and few use a 2-point, 'true/false' scoring approach. The fewer the number of scoring categories within the range of 2–10, the lower the reliability will be, especially between 2 and 5 categories (Streiner and Norman 1998). Although this argues for using between five and seven response categories, a major problem is that raters seldom use the extreme positions, and tend to score in the middle range. This may result in a loss of discriminative power. For a rating scale it is important to discriminate 'cases' from 'noncases', or between 'at risk' versus 'low-risk' children.

Composition of scales

There are two major approaches to combining a number of individual problem items to assess an underlying aspect of functioning.

Empirical versus the nosological approach

The first is the empirical-quantitative approach, which employs multivariate statistical techniques, such as factor analysis or principal components analysis. They are applied to the scores on the problem items to identify sets of problems that tend to occur together. These co-occurring items make up syndromes. Each syndrome can be quantified by summing the scores of the items that compose the syndrome. This approach can be described as working 'from the ground up', because it starts with empirical data derived from informants who describe the behavior of representative samples of children, without assumptions about whether or not the syndrome reflects diagnostic categories from standard nosological systems.

It is not always clear from the description of the derivation of scales listed in the main text whether the authors used general population samples or clinical samples to compute their syndrome scales.

It remains a matter of controversy what kind of samples is needed to create the scales. Some use clinical samples as the data source for the multivariate analyses of syndrome scales, because clinical samples yield items with frequencies high enough to be retained in reliable factor analysis or principal component analysis. Also, the use of clinical samples will result in scales that relate to aggregations of problems as encountered in clinical practice. Others, especially those who use rating scales in general population samples, argue that syndrome scales should be based on data derived from general population samples, because the factor structure should reflect the underlying structure of problems in the samples to be studied. Before using a factor structure in samples that are essentially different from the ones from which the factor structure was derived, it is important to test the applicability of the factor structure.

The second approach is to take the diagnostic categories of one of the two international nosological systems, the fourth edition of the American Psychiatric Association's (1994) *Diagnostic and Statistical Manual of Mental Disorders (DSM-IV)* and the World Health Organization's (1992) *International Classification of Diseases (ICD)*, as the basis for the syndromes that can be scored with the rating scale. The DSM and ICD categories are formed on the basis of negotiations among panels of experts, who selected the target disorders and the criteria for defining them. This approach can be described as working 'from the top down', because it starts with assumptions about which disorders exist and about how to identify individuals who might have them.

Although the empirical and nosological approaches converge, they do not converge to a degree that one approach can replace the other. Both the empirical and nosological approaches to the derivation of syndrome scales have advantages and disadvantages.

The advantage of the empirical approach is that it does not start from assumptions about the disorders that exist. Because we still lack empirical evidence about the true nature and boundaries of child/adolescent psychiatric disorders, the empirical approach can help to improve existing knowledge about nosology. Since the empirical approach starts with data derived from representative samples of children and adolescents, the intrinsic validity of this procedure is appealing. However, a disadvantage of the empirical approach is that the empirically based syndrome scales vary as a function of the item content, the number of items, the statistical technique that was used to compute the syndromes, and the samples that

were used to derive the data. As a consequence, the content and the number of scales differ across the different instruments. Although there is convergence between the scales across different instruments, they do not converge to a degree that one set of scales can replace the other.

An advantage of the nosological approach is that despite the lack of validity of most DSM and ICD diagnostic categories, they represent a system that is widely accepted. This facilitates communication across researchers and clinicians.

Instead of disregarding one approach for the other, we hold the view that both approaches are needed, and that combining both approaches by adding information from one approach that is not captured by the other, may aid in increasing our knowledge of psychopathology.

Overall index of dysfunction

So far we have discussed the approaches to determine syndrome scales that can be scored from individual problem scores. For some purposes, it is not necessary to use syndrome scales; for instance, when we only want to estimate whether or not an individual should be regarded as disordered or not. In that case we need an indication of the individual's overall level of dysfunction.

The sum of the problem scores, the total problem score, usually serves as a general indicator of the overall level of psychopathology. Because the length of the total problem scale is much greater than that of the syndrome scales, the reliability of the total problem scale usually is greater than that of most of the syndrome scales. However, this gain in reliability is often at the expense of a reduction in validity as a result of a lack of differentiation. Most rating scales have the option to compute a total problem score in addition to computing syndrome scores.

Externalizing and internalizing scales

It is also possible that users need a measure of the child's or adolescent's problem behavior on a level of precision that is intermediate between the fine grained syndrome level and the crude total problem score. For those purposes, a number of instruments use two broad band groupings of syndromes called 'externalizing' and 'internalizing'. When problems are externalized, this reflects conflicts with other people and their expectations of the child or adolescent, whereas internalizing a problem reflects internal distress. The externalizing and internalizing groupings are usually determined through second order factor analyses of the correlations among the syndrome scale scores.

Weighting of items

Some would argue that by simply adding up all of the items we will lose valuable information, since some items may be more important than others, and hence should make a larger contribution to the scale score than those that are less important. For scales that were derived through factor analyses, the analyses yield factor loadings for each item constituting the scale. The size of the factor loading indicates the relative contribution of the item to the scale. These factor loadings may be used as an index for weighting the items.

Another approach to weighting items is theoretical or clinical-intuitive. For instance, one may speculate that feeling sad and depressed, or having repetitive thoughts about dying and suicide, are more important contributors to the concept of depression than are sleeping problems or weight loss.

Differential weighting may yield greater precision; for example, in predicting outcome, especially for smaller scales. However, it is generally felt that this will contribute relatively little, except added complexity for the scorer (Streiner and Norman 1998). The greater complexity certainly is a drawback for applying differential weighting in everyday clinical practice.

Percentiles and T-scores

As described above, most rating scales can be scored on a number of subscales. The various subscales of the same instrument have different mean scores in reference samples because of differences in the number of items of each scale, and because of differences in the mean item scores. As a consequence each scale is scored on a different metric, making comparison across syndrome scales difficult. For instance, how can we compare a score of 20 on a syndrome scale measuring aggression with a scoring range between 0 and 40, with a score of 10 on a syndrome scale measuring depression with a scoring range between 0 and 20? Because both scales are measured on different yardsticks this is not possible without transforming the raw scores into scores that have a similar metric.

One approach is the use of *percentiles*. A percentile is the percentage of individuals who score below a certain value. The lowest value is the 0th percentile; the highest value is the 99th percentile. Well-known examples in medicine are the height and weight charts used to assess the physical development of children. Percentiles can be computed on the basis of questionnaire scores for a representative sample of children who are ranked from the highest to the lowest score. In most cases this will be a general population sample, or a sample of 'normal' children, usually a general population sample with the

exclusion of children known to have a behavioral/ emotional problem, such as children referred for mental health services. It is also possible to use referred samples or samples of clinical children with one specific disorder such as autism. The advantage of percentiles is that they are easy to interpret. For instance, if a boy received a score on the aggression scale corresponding with the 90th percentile based on the cumulative frequency distribution of scores in a normative sample of boys in the same age range, this means that only 10% of normal boys of the same age obtained higher aggression scores.

A second approach to transforming scores into those that can be compared across scales with different metrics is the use of *T-scores*. A T-score is a score with a mean of 50 and a standard deviation of 10. A T-score of 50 will correspond with the 50th percentile. The advantage of both percentiles and T-scores is that they allow us to determine where an individual's score stands in relation to scores of individuals of the same sex and age. The advantage of T-scores over percentiles is that, since they are more or less normally distributed, they allow us to use parametric statistics, and therefore means and standard deviations can be computed. Of course, the utility of both percentiles and T-scores depends on the size and how representative of the reference samples they are.

Psychometric properties of rating scales

Reliability

Any measurement is affected by a certain amount of error, both random and systematic. The ratio of variability between subjects, or true score variation, to the total measurement variability (the sum of subject variability, random error and systematic error) is called reliability. In practice, reliability refers to the replicability of measurement.

When rating scales are self-administered by the parent, teacher, or adolescent him- or herself, it is important to know to which degree the same informants provide similar results on different occasions. The time intervals used for assessing the *test–retest reliability* should be short enough to expect that the subject's behavior did not change. In the case of teachers as informants it is possible to assess the level of agreement between scores obtained from one teacher to another teacher or teacher's aide. This type of reliability is called *inter-rater reliability*.

Because parents are such a central source of information on their child's functioning, it also helpful to know the degree of agreement between scores from fathers and mothers. Since reliability involves variation in assessments of the same phenomena, *inter-parent agreement* should not be treated as a reliability measure. Ratings by mothers and fathers are based on somewhat different samples of the child's behavior. Consequently inter-parent agreement is not expected to be as high as test–retest or inter-interviewer reliability.

As scores obtained through repeated measurements can be affected both by their rank ordering and by differences in magnitude, it is important that reliability measures reflect both these factors. Pearson correlation coefficients are often used as reliability measure but are only affected by differences in rank ordering of the correlated scores, whereas T-tests for assessing the difference between mean scores are only affected by differences between the magnitudes of scores. A measure that is affected both by differences in the rank ordering and the magnitude of scores is the *intraclass correlation coefficient* (ICC; Shrout and Fleiss 1979). When evaluating the psychometric qualities of an instrument, it is important to be aware of the kind of reliability measure that is reported.

Reliability is often treated as an intrinsic characteristic of a measure. This is not true. Reliability of a measure is highly linked to the population to which the measure is applied, and to the procedure with which the reliability is tested.

For most rating scales listed in the main text, data on test–retest reliability are reported, and where appropriate data on inter-rater reliability, or inter-parent agreement. Reliability measures for these instruments are usually favorable for broad measures such as total problem scores. For some subscales reliability may be lower and, in fact, problematic in some instances. The data is too complex to present here. Rather, we would like to stress the importance of the user carefully evaluating the reliability of the instrument for the particular purpose for which it is intended to be used.

A somewhat different measure, also referred to as reliability, is the instrument's index of *internal consistency*, often presented as coefficient alpha, or Cronbach's alpha (Schmitt 1996). Alpha is a function of the interrelatedness of the items in a test. Internal consistency does not tell us anything about the degree to which an instrument will give us the same results over different occasions such as the reliability measures discussed so far. However, most authors of the rating scales listed in the main text report internal consistencies by convention and, in all instances, the internal consistencies are very high. In most instances it was found that the smaller the scale, the smaller the internal consistency.

Validity

Validity refers to the degree an instrument measures what it is designed to measure. The most basic form of validity is *content validity*. Content validity is strongly related to the choice of items. If the aim was to design a scale that would cover DSM-IV categories and the scale consists of questions that are highly compatible to DSM-IV criteria, then the content validity will be high. The limits of the validity of a scale using items covering DSM-IV categories will then be determined by the validity of the DSM-IV categories.

If the aim was to design a scale that taps a broad range of items that are of clinical concern to parents and mental health workers, the items of the instrument should discriminate between clinically referred and non-referred children and adolescents (a criterion that can also be used to determine criterion related validity). Consequently, items that do not discriminate between clinically referred and non-referred children and adolescents are often omitted from the scoring or from subsequent versions of an instrument.

Construct validity reflects the fact that, in the field of psychopathology, we deal with variables that are abstract and that cannot be easily operationally defined as can some physical variables. Anxiety, depression, and even conduct problems all are supposed to have underlying factors referred to as hypothetical constructs. In statistical language this inferred variable is called 'latent variable'. There is no single test that can establish an instrument's construct validity. Construct validation is an ongoing process of interrelated procedures through which we try to learn more about a certain construct. These procedures can be tests that determine the relationship of an instrument's syndromes with numerous other variables such as etiological, prognostic, or outcome variables or responses to treatment. In this way, each new study can strengthen what Cronbach and Meehl (1955) called the 'nomological network' of interrelated procedures intended to reflect the underlying construct.

Instruments that have been used in many studies have the advantage that there are many data potentially confirming the validity of the syndromes.

Another way to determine the construct validity is to compare the instrument to other instruments that are intended to measure similar constructs. This is sometimes called *concurrent validity*. For instance, the correlations between the scales of one instrument with those of another can be computed. This raises the question of why this should be done. If a good criterion measure already exists, why then bother about another instrument that intends to measure the same constructs? The most prevalent reason why this is done is because the instrument used as the criterion is too long or expensive. This may be the case when a brief and inexpensive rating scale is compared with a much more time consuming and expensive clinical interview.

Criterion related validity refers to the relationship of a measure to another measure that is regarded as the 'gold standard'. For brief scales, this type of validity can be called *predictive validity*. The external reference criterion for a brief rating scale usually takes the form of a comprehensive clinical diagnostic evaluation that definitively establishes the presence or absence of the index condition. However, given the present state of the art in the field of child and adolescent psychopathology, there is no infallible criterion that can serve as the gold standard for the presence or absence of most disorders, and the boundaries between them.

One way to test the criterion related validity of a rating scale is to test the relationship between the questionnaire scale scores and DSM diagnoses derived from standardized interviews, or with DSM diagnoses derived through unstandardized clinical procedures. Because there is little empirical ground for assuming that one approach is intrinsically superior to the other, in fact these studies tested the concurrent validity between the questionnaire and the psychiatric interview. This view is supported by a study by Boyle et al. (1997) who compared the associations of a rating scale (the Ontario Child Health Study scales) with a psychiatric interview (the revised version of the Diagnostic Interview for Children and Adolescents; DICA) to external validators. They concluded that differences in validity between the two assessment procedures were small, and where present they even showed a somewhat better performance for the rating scale than for the interview.

Referral status is used for many rating scales to test the criterion related validity by testing the ability of an instrument to discriminate between children and adolescents who are referred for mental health services and those who are non-referred. Referral status is not an infallible morbidity criterion either, because some children and adolescents are referred for other reasons than being truly disordered. Conversely, it is known that many disordered children and adolescents in the general population do not receive professional help for their problems. When an instrument is tested against referral status as the criterion, this may result in an underestimate of the ability to discriminate between disordered and normal children or adolescents.

Scoring procedures and interpretation

The scoring procedures and the interpretation of the results of a rating scale should be easy to follow and understandable. Most rating scales have scoring forms or graphic displays that describe the scores relative to the norms. Computerized scoring and profile printouts in graphic form have many advantages. Scoring profiles that use reference data make it possible to graphically display

an individual's scores in relation to scores of reference individuals of the same sex and age. When the syndrome scale scores of an instrument are converted to T-scores, scales with different metrics can be easily compared and displayed on the same profile.

There is a certain pressure to present and interpret the scores of rating scales in a 'user friendly' way, especially in clinical settings. Ready made or 'canned' interpretations of the scores mechanically applied to each case bear the risk of losing essential information and of misinterpretation. It is the clinician's or researcher's task to synthesize information from diverse sources into optimal interpretations. This implies that the clinician or researcher is aware of the strengths and weaknesses of the assessment procedures that are used. Rating scales are developed to assist in determining the likelihood that the subject does or does not have the specific problem the instrument is designed to identify. 'Use for any other purpose (e.g. assigning a diagnosis based solely on the instrument's results...) only serves to undermine the integrity of the instrument...' (Maruish 1999).

Translation

There is a growing need for translations of psychometrically sound rating scales, mostly from English into other languages. This need comes from researchers and clinicians in various countries but also from researchers and clinicians who work in major metropolitan areas having a multi-ethnic, multi-language character.

There are no generally accepted guidelines for gauging the adequacy of translation, although there is an increasing awareness of the many difficulties in the faithful translation of instruments (Canino and Bravo 1999; Streiner and Norman 1998; Weisz and Eastman 1995). The translation procedure should result in a version that is equivalent with respect to the meaning of the items. This is done through a translation-back-translation procedure, which should preferably be carried out by two different translators who are bilingual and who are knowledgeable about the content area. However, this may result in a translation with a slightly different meaning than the original item. To ensure optimal accuracy in translations, some authors advice to repeat the translation-back-translation procedure, sometimes several times (Weisz and Eastman 1995), whereas others emphasize the importance of field testing (Canino and Bravo 1999). However, even very accurate translations may result in linguistic nuances that need explicit reporting.

Accurate translation is the first step towards using an existing instrument in different cultural settings. The second step is the testing of the instrument's psychometric properties in these other contexts, including its reliability and validity. In particular, in case empirically derived syndromes are used, the factorial structure needs to be determined and compared across different cultural settings. The third step is the derivation of reference scores, both in representative normative and clinical samples. The last step is the testing whether scores are comparable across different populations or cultures.

For a few scales (e.g. Achenbach and Rescorla 1999; Conners 1997) information on the presence and the quality of versions in other languages is available, but for the majority of scales this is not the case. Because systematic information on translations and local norms was lacking for the majority of scales, we have omitted this information in this edition. Hopefully it will be possible to include this important information in a next edition.

Advantages and disadvantages of rating scales

One of the great advantages of rating scales over clinical interviews is that they can be applied in a flexible, easy to administer and economic way. Administration time usually is modest. Most rating scales listed in this book will take between 10 and 20 minutes to be completed. They can be administered in various locations such as home, school or (mental) health settings. Rating scales are also characterized by a great flexibility in the way they can be administered: in person, by telephone or by mail. Administration can be facilitated by using computer assisted client entry programs. Some rating scales have a computer assisted client entry program.

Rating scales need not be administered by expensive clinically trained professionals. These characteristics make it possible to obtain uniform data across different populations and different settings in a relatively easy and economical way. For example, rating scales can be routinely administered in (mental) health settings at intake, or can be used in large scale epidemiological surveys. This is needed to obtain reference data on normal as well as clinically referred children and adolescents.

Thanks to their practicality, a number of rating scales have a large amount of data on reliability and validity. This gives us detailed information on the variation that can typically be expected.

Rating scales have a number of disadvantages too, some of which are shared by other measurement procedures as well. Rating scales are limited to the informant's perspective. Characteristics of the informant and the tendency toward response biases are sources of variation in ratings. Rating scales are limited to the structured scores

for standardized items. Information that may be relevant but that is not covered by the items of the scale may be missed. It is not possible to explore the informant's responses and subjective experiences, nor is it possible to observe behavior directly. Misunderstandings and ambiguous answers that may be clarified in a clinical interview are missed when using questionnaires. Also slight changes in the wording of instructions, or the wording of the items themselves, may have large effects that limit comparability (e.g. Woodward et al. 1989).

Many of the above mentioned problems can be prevented by unambiguous wording of items and instructions. For instance, before having a respondent complete a rating scale, we must have an indication about the respondent's reading skills.

Measures of accuracy of rating scales

Rating scales applied to populations not known to have psychiatric conditions can be regarded as *screening tests*, whereas the same questionnaires applied to populations known to have symptoms can be termed *diagnostic tests* (Weiss 1998). The underlying rationale for the use of a test is identical for both screening and diagnostic tests. The rationale is that, among individuals to whom the test is administered, the monetary, physical and psychological costs of the condition along with the cost of the test and the errors that arise when the test does not classify individuals accurately, will be exceeded by the costs of the condition, had the test not been done.

Sensitivity and specificity

The usefulness of a test depends on its accuracy. This can be assessed in several different ways: by sensitivity, specificity, positive and negative prediction. Sensitivity and specificity do not reflect an intrinsic quality of a test. They are not absolute values. Sensitivity and specificity will vary with the samples on which they were based and with the critical values chosen.

Robins (1985) illustrated how the sensitivity of a test for the presence of a psychiatric disorder was higher in a patient sample than in a general population sample. Such tests usually detect severe cases more readily than mild ones. In a patient sample with many severe cases, the sensitivity of a test for detecting disorder will be higher than in a general population sample containing the whole range of possible severities. The specificity of a test for the presence of disorder will be higher in general population samples than in patient samples. Incorrect classification of those without a disorder as cases will be lowest for individuals with none or very few problems and highest for individuals who score just below the threshold between having a disorder and not. In a general population sample with a large proportion of individuals with no or very few problems, the specificity of a test will be higher than in a patient sample with more individuals scoring just below the threshold for disorder.

Rating scales cannot serve as absolute tests of the presence or absence of a disorder. The frequency distributions of problem scores derived from rating scales completed for normal and disordered children or adolescents show considerable overlap. Measurements of child/adolescent psychopathology do not result in a clear distinction between disordered and nondisordered individuals, because the polygenetic nature of most disorders and the heterogeneous environments result in continuously distributed phenotypes, and because the measurements of the phenotypes are imperfect. As a result there are no cut-off points for questionnaires that perfectly separate disordered from nondisordered individuals. In other words there are no questionnaires with both perfect (100%) sensitivity and specificity.

Cut-off points are chosen by making compromises among several considerations. Any cut-off point that is chosen is a trade off between sensitivity and specificity. Sensitivity and specificity vary with the cut-off point chosen and, because both values are inversely related, sensitivity can only be increased at the expense of specificity, and specificity can only be increased at the expense of sensitivity.

The relationship between sensitivity and specificity can also be expressed by a so called Receiver Operating Characteristic (ROC) curve. The ROC curve is constructed by plotting the sensitivity on the vertical axis, against the false positive rate (100-specificity) on the horizontal axis. The use of ROC curves has two advantages. The first is that the curve readily shows the trade off between sensitivity and specificity, which makes it easier to determine the optimal scoring range for choosing the cut-off point that matches the aims of the user best. Secondly, the area under the curve (AUC) can be computed and used as an index for the criterion related validity of a test. The AUC can be conceptualized as the probability of correctly identifying a randomly chosen pair of individuals (one who has the disorder, one who does not). The AUC ranges between 0.5 – which indicates that the test does not add to the chance probability of correctly classifying individuals – and 1.0, which would indicate a perfect test. The AUC enables us to compare the discriminative power of different rating scales (e.g. Kresanov et al. 1998).

The accuracy of a test can also be expressed as the extent to which being categorized as 'test positive' or 'test negative' actually predicts the presence of the disorder. This may be an important approach for individual children and adolescents in determining the probability that an individual has a certain disorder, given the results of a test.

Predictive value is influenced by prevalence. In a sample with relatively few disordered individuals, the positive predictive value (PV+) of even a very specific test will be low, indicating that a 'positive' result of the test will yield many false positives. If the same test will be used in a sample with a much higher prevalence, the PV+ will be much higher. The problem of low base rates does not affect the positive predictive and the negative predictive values equally. It is only the positive predictive value which is substantially affected by low base rates. This is especially the case when base rates drop under 1%. This makes screening for very rare disorders such as autism using rating scales in community settings unattractive.

Although the problem of low base rates for predicting rare conditions, even with highly valid tests, was observed long ago (Meehl and Rosen 1955), Clark and Harrington (1999) showed that few child mental health professionals who regularly use questionnaires to screen for mental disorders were aware of this problem.

A technique that can be used to overcome low base rates problems is *sequential screening* (Derogatis and Lynn 1998). With this method two different rating scales are used in two phases. In the first phase, a screening procedure is applied with the main aim being to correctly identify individuals who do not have the condition, and eliminate them for the second phase sample. This results in an enriched sample with a much higher prevalence of the condition. In the second phase, a rating scale with an equal or superior sensitivity will be used, and because the base rate of the condition in the second phase sample is much higher, the PV+ of the test will also be higher, and the misclassification of normal individuals as being disordered will be lower. The predictive value of a test is also influenced by the chosen cut-off point.

For some rating scales in the main text, the authors specify the sensitivity and specificity. They usually are satisfactory and in the same range as rating scales for adult psychiatric disorders. However, the relativistic nature of these measures makes it imperative for the potential user to judge these values against the background of the specific purposes for which the rating scale is intended.

Epidemiological application of screening procedures

There are two main areas of application of screening procedures: (i) screening for public health and epidemiological purposes, and (ii) screening procedures for service settings.

The main difference between the two areas of application is that for epidemiological purposes we often need assessments of individuals that do not need the involvement of a professional who has responsibility for the individual. The prevalence of a disorder in a community sample, for instance, or the need for help, can de determined by assessments of individuals without the direct involvement of a health professional. In contrast, screening procedures that are used in service settings, such as in pediatric care, need the involvement of a professional who is qualified to make decisions and who is already responsible for the individual.

Epidemiology, with its emphasis on large scale measurements, has an evident need for assessment procedures that are accurate, practical and economical. When the first child psychiatric epidemiological studies were planned, the lack of such assessment procedures was the driving force for developing the first generation of brief rating scales.

Multistage/multimethod sampling

Epidemiological measures for large scale descriptive or etiological studies usually need to be brief and inexpensive. Especially when investigating conditions with low base rates, it is problematic to use elaborate procedures to assess many individuals who do not have a disorder. Therefore, it is advantageous to use a multistage sampling approach. We described a two-stage sampling approach using rating scales in each stage in the paragraph where we described how to overcome the problem of low base rates. A procedure that is often used in epidemiological studies is the multistage/multimethod approach, a combination of the psychometric and clinical approaches (Dohrenwend and Dohrenwend 1982; Verhulst and Koot 1992).

In stage 1 a rating scale is applied to the total sample in which the base rate of a disorder is relatively low. Individuals with high problem scores are designated cases or 'screen positives'. All others are designated noncases or 'screen negatives'.

In stage 2, all 'screen positives' and a random sample of the 'screen negatives' from stage 1 are assessed using more elaborate procedures such as a clinical interview. The results of the interviews will confirm or disconfirm 'caseness' as determined in stage 1. Confirmation of classification will result in 'true positives' and 'true negatives', disconfirmation will result in 'false positives' and 'false negatives'.

For some purposes this two-stage approach may be sufficient. However, if we aim for greater precision, we can introduce a third assessment procedure preferably using other indices of malfunctioning. This may be a measure of social competence, a measure of global functioning, or some alternative method such as the use of records. Usually stage 3 assessments aim at obtaining a much more complete picture of an individual's functioning. Stage 3 assessments can be applied to the whole stage 2 sample, or only to the 'false negatives' and 'false positives' to classify individuals.

The rating scales used in stage 1 can be used in different ways to classify individuals. The first is to use the total problem score as a global index of dysfunction and to identify individuals who score above the cut-off point. Most generic rating scales, however, have the option to include specific syndrome scales in the selection of individuals. It is possible to identify individuals who score above the cut-off point of any of the syndrome scales that can be scored from the generic rating scale. This can be an advantage because some individuals, who score above the cut-off point of a specific syndrome scale, may score below the cut-off point for the total problem score. The reverse may also be true. Individuals who score above the cut-off point for the total problem score need not reach the cut-off point for any of the specific syndrome scales. Because selection of individuals based solely on one strategy (either the total problem score or the syndrome scales) may miss cases that would have been identified by the other strategy, it may be an advantage to combine both approaches. Individuals can then be selected for further assessment who score above the cut-off point on *either* the total problem score *or* on any of the syndrome scales, or *both*. When both the total problem score and the syndrome scales are used to select high scoring individuals, not only will the number of cases identified by the procedure be increased (a higher sensitivity), but also the number of normal individuals misclassified as disordered (lower specificity). This need not be a problem if we aim at a higher specificity in the stage 2 assessment.

Specific questionnaires, generic questionnaires, or both?

When we are interested in only one disorder, for instance depression, it is possible to use a brief questionnaire in stage 1 that is focussed on the condition we are interested in. Individuals who score high on this depression questionnaire and a random sample of the low scoring subjects will be selected for stage 2 assessments. However, if we choose a specific selection strategy in stage 1, it is important that the stage 2 assessments cover a much broader range of psychopathology. Otherwise we will miss problems that are associated with depression (for instance, conduct problems) and that are strongly related to factors such as outcome or therapeutic effect. Consider as an example an outcome study on children with attention deficit hyperactivity disorder (ADHD) in which only ratings on ADHD and not on conduct problems were obtained. With such an approach, information on a strong determinant for poor outcome would be overlooked. The broader stage 2 assessment can either be done with a generic rating scale or an interview that covers a wide range of psychopathology.

Multiple specific questionnaires or one generic questionnaire?

A question that may arise is whether it is better to use one generic rating scale or multiple specific rating scales at the initial stage of assessment. As discussed above, most generic rating scales have the option of using the total problem score, the specific syndrome scales, or both to score each individual. A disadvantage of using multiple instruments that specifically assess one area such as depression, anxiety, or hyperactivity is that each instrument has its own metric and norms, making comparisons difficult, and that there may be considerable overlap in the items across the various instruments.

Combining information from multiple informants

So far we have discussed the application of multiple stages and multiple methods of assessment in screening. The issue of multiple informants has not yet been considered. Because the agreement between different sources (e.g. parents, teachers, adolescents' self-reports) is rather low, there is little overlap in individuals identified by different informants in screening procedures. If the initial screening of a population is based on information from one informant only, and the broader and more individualized assessments in the next stage is based on multiple informants (e.g. clinical parent and child interview, teacher information) the accuracy of the initial screening procedure will be low. The addition of other screening sources including teacher or adolescents' self-report information will enhance the accuracy of the procedure. Therefore, it is important to combine information from different informants.

A number of strategies can be employed to combine information from different informants if the results are treated in a categorical way (Institute of Medicine 1989), including:

- giving value to any positive rating, regardless of the informant;
- only giving value to ratings scored positively by more than one informant; and
- giving priority to one informant for certain types of problems.

The use of multiple sources of information at the same time can be regarded as parallel testing. Each strategy for combining the results from multiple tests has its consequences for the sensitivity and specificity of the assessment procedure. If we accept any positive result, the

sensitivity of the procedure will be higher than when all tests need to be positive. The more restrictive the criterion, the lower the sensitivity will be, and the more disturbed the individuals who are selected.

There is yet another way to combine information from different informants if we treat the data from rating scales as continuous scores. A problem with combining scores derived from different informants is that the scores on the different versions of an instrument have different metrics. We can overcome this problem by transforming the scores for each version into standard scores (z-scores). Z-scores have a mean of 0 and a standard deviation of 1. It is now possible to compute each individual's mean z-score across the three versions of the rating scale in our example. Next we can compute the frequency distribution of the mean z-scores for the sample. By applying a cut-off point to this frequency distribution, we can determine the individuals who score above this cut-off point and who may be selected for further evaluation (Verhulst et al. 1997).

Clinical applications of rating scales

The application of rating scales need not only to be confined to community samples. Rating scales can also be applied to populations known to have high levels of psychiatric morbidity, including children and adolescents in the mental health care system, the primary health care system, pediatric care, (special) schools, the juvenile justice system, or facilities for mentally retarded children and adolescents.

Many countries have financial constraints or other limitations to the services that can be provided to children and adolescents with mental health problems. It is therefore essential that the professional's valuable time is not being wasted in lengthy and inefficient assessment procedures, or in interventions that do not fit the problem.

A primary task of mental health professionals working with children and adolescents is to assess individuals who have behavioral/emotional problems. Another primary task is to make decisions how children and adolescents who have problems can be helped best. To perform these tasks in an efficient way, numerous decisions have to be made.

If parents contact a clinic about their child's behavior, the first decision that needs to be made is whether the parents' report indicates a severe enough problem to warrant referral to the clinic for further evaluation. It is also important to decide whether the clinic is the most appropriate setting for evaluating the problem, or whether the child and the parents should be referred to another facility.

If the decision is made that the child should be assessed in the clinic, then other decisions have to be made, including what diagnostic assessment data should be obtained, what type of treatment should be provided, what is the duration of the treatment, how much should the child's functioning improve, and what should be done after treatment?

Clinical practice can benefit from a standardized approach to the numerous decisions that need to be made from case to case. When we base decisions on explicit rules that follow assessment data on individual cases, we may improve our methods of helping children and adolescents. The process from first contact of a parent with the clinic to the termination of treatment consists of a chain of decisions. Assessment data need to be tailored to the specific needs for each step that precedes a decision. This process can be called 'triage', a term used in wartime to indicate the assignment of degrees of urgency to decide the order of treatment.

Rating scales can play a useful role in this process. For example, rating scales can play a role at the beginning of the referral process by mailing them to parents, teachers or adolescents themselves. We have emphasized earlier that rating scales cannot and should not be used to replace comprehensive diagnostic case formulation, which needs to be based on a multitude of information, including psychiatric parent and child interviews, psychological and physical test data, and information on social competence. Rating scale data (for instance teacher data) can serve as one source of the full evaluation, but they can also assist,

together with information on the referral complaint, in assigning cases to certain programs, or certain mental health professionals.

Once a comprehensive case formulation is made, rating scale data can assist in selecting certain targets for intervention. There is evidence that several types of interventions are effective under research conditions, but that these positive effects cannot be repeated under typical clinical conditions (Weisz et al. 1992). If standardized assessments to identify the target problems needed to match the most appropriate treatment are carried out for every case, and this information is then accumulated, it may be possible to better identify those children and adolescents that resemble those who benefited most from a certain intervention. By monitoring the effects of interventions, it may be possible to change the practice of assigning cases to certain interventions, or to alter the interventions that are provided. Rating scales can be valuable for monitoring the effects of interventions by their readministration.

Lastly, rating scales can be used to evaluate the outcomes of interventions. In clinical settings outcome evaluations can be done on a regular basis. If certain types of cases or interventions have poor outcomes, this may result in changes in practice. In pediatric practice it is common to evaluate chronic patients on a regular basis (e.g. patients with diabetes, chronic respiratory disease, epilepsy, etc.). Also, the field of child and adolescent

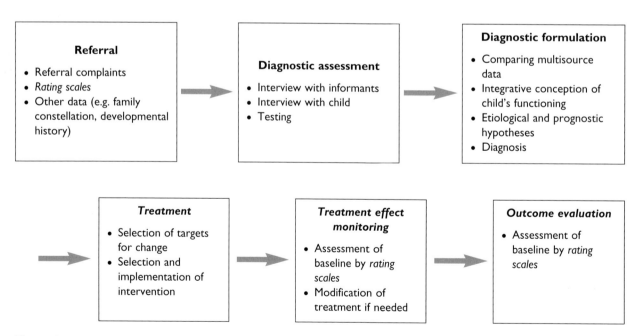

Figure 1

Steps in the clinical process. Rating scales (printed in italic in the figure) can be used as one of many sources of information to assess a child's problems, to monitor treatment effects, to evaluate (long-term) outcome and to aid the clinician in making decisions.

psychiatry can benefit from evaluating the outcomes of interventions and to relate that to the type and the duration of the care that had been provided.

Figure 1 presents an overview of the typical sequence of clinical data gathering, diagnostic formulation and case management. This flowchart, which was adapted from an overview of empirically based assessment procedures by Achenbach and McConaughy (1997), shows where in the clinical process rating scales can be used next to the other assessment procedures that are used in the various steps the clinician and patient go through after the patient is referred for mental health services. The clinician has the task of integrating the multitude of data derived from multiple sources of information, including information derived from rating scales. Based on the often conflicting information, the clinician has to make decisions as to what type of treatment will be best for a particular child's problems. Rating scales can especially be helpful as part of the assessment process and for monitoring treatment effects and to evaluate (long-term) outcome.

Criteria for selecting a rating scale

There are many similarities between the different rating scales. Some scales cover roughly similar areas, most have evidence of adequate reliability and validity, most are user-friendly and most can be scored in a comprehensive way. However, there are also some differences that may be relevant for some purposes. Answering the following questions may aid in making a choice of which scale to use.

1. Do I need multiple informants? Some scales have versions for parents, teachers and self-reports, whereas other scales only have versions for one informant.
2. Do I need a rating scale for early assessment or screening, or do I need one for more extensive evaluation, and will the instrument be completed for one individual or for many individuals by the same informant (for instance all children in one classroom by one teacher)? Most scales take between 10 and 20 minutes to complete, but there are also scales that take only a few minutes to complete.
3. Do I need to assess problems only, or do I need to assess competence as well. Some scales have competence or adaptive functioning items as well as problem items.
4. Do I want to obtain ratings that can be scored on DSM-oriented scales, on empirically derived scales, or on both?
5. Are translations of the instrument available in the languages that I need? The availability of scales in different languages may not be only an advantage for

cross-cultural research but also for the assessment of children from different cultures living in our present day pluriform societies.

6. Are there local norms available for the assessment scale?
7. Do I want to compare my findings with those from others? Of course, the most widely used instruments have the most well-documented and published findings with which new findings can be compared.

References

Achenbach TM, Rescorla LE. Mental Health Practitioners' Guide for the Achenbach System of Empirically Based Assessment (ASEBA). Burlington, VT: University of Vermont Department of Psychiatry, 1999.

Achenbach TM, McConaughy SH, Howell CT. Child /adolescent behavioral and emotional problems: Implication of cross-informant correlations for situational specificity. Psychol Bull 1987; 101: 213–32.

American Psychiatric Association. Diagnostic and Statistical Manual of Mental Disorders, 4th edn. Washington DC: American Psychiatric Association, 1994.

Boyle MH, Offord DR, Racine YA, Szatmari P, Sanford M, Fleming JE. Interview versus checklists: adequacy for clarifying childhood psychiatric disorder based on parent reports. Arch Gen Psychiatr 1997; 54: 793–9.

Canino G, Bravo M. The translation and adaptation of diagnostic instruments for cross-cultural use. In: Shaffer D, Lucas CP, Richters JE. Diagnostic Assessment in Child and Adolescent Psychopathology. New York, NY: The Guilford Press, 1999.

Clark A, Harrington R. On diagnosing rare disorders rarely: appropriate use of rating scales. J Child Psychol Psychiatr 1998; 40: 287–90.

Conners CK. Conners' Rating Scales – Revised Technical Manual. North Tonawanda, New York: Multi Health Systems, 1997.

Cronbach LJ, Meehl PE. Construct validity in psychological tests. Psychol Bull 1955; 52: 281–302.

Derogatis LR, Lynn LL. Psychological tests in screening for psychiatric disorder. In: Maruish ME (editor). The use of psychological testing for treatment planning and outcomes assessment, 2nd edn. Mahwah, NJ: Lawrence Erlbaum, 1998.

Dohrenwend BP, Dohrendwend BS. Perspectives on the past and future of psychiatric epidemiology. Am J Publ Health 1982; 72: 1271–9.

Institute of Medicine. Research on children and adolescents with mental, behavioral and development disorders: Mobilizing a national initiative. Washington DC: National Academy Press, 1989.

Jensen PS, Rubio-Stipec M, Canino G, Bird HR, Dulcan M, Schwab-Stone ME, Lahey BB. Parent and child contributions to diagnosis of mental disorder: Are both informants always necessary? J Am Acad Child Adolescent Psychiatr 1999; 38: 1569–79.

Kresanov K, Tuominen J, Piha J, Almqvist F. Validity of child psychiatric screening methods. Eur Child Adolescent Psychiatr 1998; 7: 85–95.

Maruish ME. The use of psychological testing for treatment planning and outcomes assessment, 2nd edn. Mahwah, NJ: Lawrence Erlbaum associates, 1999.

Meehl PE, Rosen A. Antecedent probability and the efficiency of psychometric signs, patterns, or cutting scores. Psychol Bull 1955; 52: 194–216.

Robins LN. Epidemiology: reflections on testing the validity of psychiatric interviews. Arch Gen Psychiatr 1985; 42: 918–24.

Schachar R, Rutter M, Smith A. The characteristics of situationally and pervasively hyperactive children: implications for syndrome definition. J Child Psychol Psychiatr 1981; 22: 375–92.

Schmitt N. Uses and abuses of coefficient alpha. Psychol Assess 1996; 8: 350–3.

Shrout PE, Fleiss JL. Intraclass correlations: uses in assessing rater reliability. Psychol Bull 1979; 86: 420–8.

Streiner DL, Norman GR. Health Measurement scales: a practical guide to their development and use. Oxford: Oxford University Press, 1998.

Verhulst FC, Koot HM. Child Psychiatric Epidemiology. Newbury Park, CA: Sage Publications, 1992.

Verhulst FC, Dekker M, Van der Ende J. Parent, teacher and self-reports as predictors of signs of disturbance in adolescents: whose information carries the most weight? Acta Psych Scand 1997; 96: 75–81.

Verhulst FC, Koot HM, Van der Ende J. Differential predictive value of parents' and teachers' reports of children's problem behaviors: a longitudinal study. J Abnormal Child Psychol 1994; 22: 531–46.

Verhulst FC, Van der Ende J, Ferdinand RF, Kasius MC. The prevalence of DSM-III-R diagnoses in a national sample of Dutch adolescents. Arch Gen Psychiatr 1997; 54: 329–36.

Weiss N. Clinical Epidemiology. In: Rothman KJ, Greenland S. Modern Epidemiology. PA: Lippincott-Raven, 1998.

Weisz JR, Eastman KL. Cross-national research on child and adolescent psychopathology. In: Verhulst FC and Koot HM. The epidemiology of child and adolescent psychopathology. Oxford: Oxford Medical Publications, 1995.

Weisz JR, Weiss B, Donenberg GR. The lab versus the clinic: effects of child and adolescent psychotherapy. Am Psychol 1992; 47: 1578–85.

Woodward CA, Thomas HB, Boyle MH, Links PS, Offord DR. Methodologic note for child epidemiological surveys: the efforts of instructions on estimates of behavior prevalence. J Child Psychol Psychiatr 1989; 30: 919–24.

World Health Organization. Mental Disorders: Glossary and guide to their classification in accordance with the tenth revision of International Classification of Diseases (10th edition). Geneva: Author, 1992

Chapter 2

General Rating Scales

Achenbach System of Empirically Based Assessment (ASEBA) – Preschool and School-Age Forms

Time Preschool forms 10–15 minutes. School-Age forms 20 minutes

Ages CBCL/1½–5: 1½–5; CBCL/6–18: 6–18; C-TRF: 1½–5; TRF: 6–18; YSR: 11–18

Time Frame CBCL/1½–5, C-TRF, TRF: last 2 months; CBCL/6–18, YSR: last 6 months

Purpose Assessment of competence, adaptive functioning, and emotional and behavioral problems.

Commentary

ASEBA forms were developed more than forty years ago and have since been updated regularly. ASEBA forms are widely used and are translated in more than 70 languages. A vast literature exists with numerous research and clinical applications.

Versions

The Achenbach System of Empirically Based Assessment (ASEBA) comprises: the Child Behavior Checklist for ages 1½–5 (CBCL/1½–5) and for ages 6–18 (CBCL/6–18) to be completed by parents or caregivers; the Caregiver-Teacher Report Form for Ages 1½–5 (C-TRF) to be completed by daycare providers or teachers; the Teacher's Report Form (TRF) to be completed by teachers of children aged 6–18, and the Youth Self-Report (YSR). In addition, ASEBA comprises the Semi-structured Clinical Interview for Children and Adolescents (SCICA) for clinicians; the Direct Observation Form (DOF) for observations in school classes, and the Test Observation Form (TOF) for observations during test taking, but these will not be discussed here.

Properties

Items The CBCL/6–18 has 20 and the YSR has 17 competence items. The TRF has 6 adaptive functioning items. The rating of competence and adaptive functioning items varies from a 4-point to 7-point format. The CBCL/1½–5 contains the Language Development Survey to be completed by parents of all children under 3, as well as by parents of children over 3 who are suspected of having language delays. Of the 310 words listed that are among the first learned by most children, the respondent

is asked to circle words that the child uses spontaneously. The CBCL/1½–5 and the C-TRF have 99, the CBCL/6–18 and TRF have 120 and the YSR has 105 emotional and behavioral problem items. In addition, the YSR has 14 socially desirable items. All problem and social desirable items are rated on a 3-point scale with responses: not true, somewhat or sometimes true, and very true or often true.

Scales Competence items of the CBCL/6–18 and the YSR can be scored on the scales Activities, Social, and (CBCL/6–18 only) School.

Factor analyses of problem item scores for children assessed in mental health and other settings as well as children from the general population with high problem scores supported eight factors that are similar for the three forms. For the Preschool Forms, the syndrome scales derived from the factor analyses are labeled Emotionally Reactive, Anxious/Depressed, Somatic Complaints, Withdrawn, Sleep Problems, Attention Problems and Aggressive Behavior, and for the School-Age Forms Anxious/Depressed, Withdrawn/Depressed, Somatic Complaints, Social Problems, Thought Problems, Attention Problems, Rule-Breaking Behavior and Aggressive Behavior. For the Preschool Forms, the first four scales, and for the School-Age Forms, the first three scales comprise problems that are mainly within the self and their sum denotes the scale Internalizing, while the last two scales comprise problems that mainly involve conflicts with others and their sum denotes the scale Externalizing. The sum of all, except the social desirable items, is the Total Problems scale.

In addition to the empirically derived problem scales, the problem items can also be scored on DSM-Oriented scales. These scales are based on experts' judgments about the correspondence between problem items and DSM-IV criteria. For the Preschool Forms, these scales are labeled Affective Problems, Anxiety Problems, Pervasive Developmental Problems, Attention Deficit/Hyperactivity Problems, Oppositional Defiant Problems, and for the School-Age Forms, these scales are labeled Affective Problems, Anxiety Problems, Somatic Problems, Attention Deficit/Hyperactivity Problems, Oppositional Defiant Problems and Conduct Problems. On the TRF only, both the syndrome scale Attention Problems and the DSM-Oriented scale Attention Deficit/Hyperactivity Problems can be divided into Inattention and Hyperactivity-Impulsivity subscales.

Reliability   Test–retest correlations over an 8-day interval for the CBCL/1½–5, the CBCL/6–18, the C-TRF, and YSR, and a 16-day interval for the TRF ranged from 0.78 to 0.93 for the social competence and adaptive functioning scales, from 0.60 to 0.96 for the syndrome scales, and from 0.62 to 0.95 for the DSM-Oriented scales.

Cronbach's alphas ranged from 0.55 to 0.79 for the social competence and adaptive functioning scales, from 0.71 to 0.97 for the syndrome scales, and from 0.67 to 0.94 for the DSM-Oriented scales.

Validity   Scales discriminate between referred and non-referred children and have significant associations with analogous scales of other instruments and with DSM criteria. ASEBA forms are widely used, therefore many studies exist that provide information about validity.

Norms   In 1999, a national survey in the USA was conducted to collect data on the ASEBA forms. For constructing norms 1753 parent-reports, 1057 self-reports, and 2319 teacher-reports were available. Raw scores were converted to normalized T-scores. Multicultural norms are being developed based on comparisons of about 30 general population samples in which ASEBA checklists were collected from all over the world.

Use   Supplementary materials are a manual describing the CBCL/6–18, YSR, and TRF, a manual describing the CBCL/1½ and C-TRF, hand-scoring profiles, a computer program for data entry and scoring, a website for data entry, scoring, and printing forms, a website for information and ordering, a bibliography listing over 6000 studies using ASEBA forms.

Key References

Achenbach TM, Rescorla LA. Manual for the ASEBA Preschool Forms & Profiles. Burlington, VT: University of Vermont, Research Center for Children, Youth, & Families, 2000.

Achenbach TM, Rescorla LA. Manual for the ASEBA School-Age Forms & Profiles. Burlington, VT: University of Vermont, Research Center for Children, Youth, & Families, 2001.

Address

ASEBA
1 South Prospect Street
Burlington, VT 05401–3456
USA
mail@aseba.org
www.aseba.org

Child Behavior Checklist for Ages 6–18 (CBCL/6–18)

Child's full name:

First   Middle   Last

Child's gender ☐ Boy ☐ Girl	Child's age	Child's ethnic group or race

Today's date Mo. ____ Day ___ Year _____	Child's birthdate Mo. ____ Day ___ Year _____

Grade in School _____   Not attending school ☐

Please fill out this form to reflect *your* view of the child's behavior even if other people might not agree. Feel free to print additional comments beside each item and in the space provided on page 2. **Be sure to answer all items.**

Parent's usual type of work, even if not working now.
(Please be specific – for example, auto mechanic, high school teacher, homemaker, laborer, lathe operator, shoe salesman, army sergeant.)

Father's type of work _____

Mother's type of work _____

This form filled out by: (print your full name)
_____

Your gender: ☐ Male   ☐ Female

Your relation to the child:

☐ Biological parent   ☐ Step parent   ☐ Grandparent

☐ Adoptive parent   ☐ Foster parent   ☐ Other (specify)

I. Please list the sports your child most likes to take part in.
For example: swimming, baseball, skating, skate boarding, bike riding, fishing, etc.

None ☐

	Compared to others of the same age, how much time does he/she spend in each?				Compared to others of the same age, how well does he/she do each one?			
	Less than average	Average	More than average	Don't know	Below average	Average	Above average	Don't know
a. _____	☐	☐	☐	☐	☐	☐	☐	☐
b. _____	☐	☐	☐	☐	☐	☐	☐	☐
c. _____	☐	☐	☐	☐	☐	☐	☐	☐

II. Please list your child's favorite hobbies activities, and games, other than sports.
For example: stamps, dolls, books, piano, crafts, cars, computing, singing, etc.)
(Do *not* include listening to radio or TV.)

None ☐

	Compared to others of the same age, about how much time does he/she spend in each?				Compared to others of the same age, how well does he/she do each one?			
	Less than average	Average	More than average	Don't know	Below average	Average	Above average	Don't know
a. _____	☐	☐	☐	☐	☐	☐	☐	☐
b. _____	☐	☐	☐	☐	☐	☐	☐	☐
c. _____	☐	☐	☐	☐	☐	☐	☐	☐

III. Please list any organizations, clubs, teams, or groups your child belongs to.

None ☐

	Compared to others of the same age, how active is he/she in each?			
	Less active	Average	More active	Don't know
a. _____	☐	☐	☐	☐
b. _____	☐	☐	☐	☐
c. _____	☐	☐	☐	☐

IV. Please list any jobs or chores your child has.
For example: paper route, babysitting, making bed, working in store, etc. (Include both paid and upaid jobs and chores.)

None ☐

	Compared to others of the same age, how well does he/she carry them out?			
	Below average	Average	Above average	Don't know
a. _____	☐	☐	☐	☐
b. _____	☐	☐	☐	☐
c. _____	☐	☐	☐	☐

V. **1. About how many close friends does your child have? (Do *not* include brothers and sisters)**

  ❑ None ❑ 1 ❑ 2 or 3 ❑ 4 or more

  2. About how many times a week does your child do things with any friends outside of regular school hours? (Do *not* include brothers and sisters)

  ❑ Less than 1 ❑ 1 or 2 ❑ 3 or more

VII. Compared to others of his/her age, how well does your child:

	Worse	Average	Better	
a. Get along with his/her brothers and sisters?	❑	❑	❑	❑ Has no brothers or sisters
b. Get along with other kids?	❑	❑	❑	
c. Behave with his/her parents?	❑	❑	❑	
d. Play and work alone?	❑	❑	❑	

VII. 1. Performance in academic subjects. **Does not attend school because** _____

Check a box for each subject that child takes	Failing	Below average	Average	Above average
a. Reading, English, or Language Arts	❑	❑	❑	❑
b. History or Social Studies	❑	❑	❑	❑
c. Arithmetic or Math	❑	❑	❑	❑
d. Science	❑	❑	❑	❑
e.	❑	❑	❑	❑
f.	❑	❑	❑	❑
g.	❑	❑	❑	❑

Other academic subjects – for example: computer courses, foreign languages, business. Do *not* include gym, shop, driver's ed., or other nonacademic subjects.

2. Does your child receive special education or remedial services or attend a special class or special school?

  ❑ No ❑ Yes – kind of services, class, or school:

3. Has your child repeated any grades? ❑ No ❑ Yes – grades and reasons:

4. Has your child had any academic or other problems in school?

  ❑ No ❑ Yes – please describe:

When did these problems start? _____

Have these problems ended? ❑ No ❑ Yes – when?

Does your child have any illness or disability (either physical or mental)? ❑ No ❑ Yes – please describe:

What concerns you most about your child?

Please describe the best things about your child.

Below is a list of items that describe children and youths. For each item that describes your child *now or within the past 6 months*, please circle the **2** if the item is *very true or often true* of your child. Circle the **I** if the item is *somewhat or sometimes true* of your child. If the item is *not true* of your child, circle the **0**. Please answer all items as well as you can, even if some do not seem to apply to your child.

0 = Not true (as far as you know)   **I = Somewhat or sometimes true**   **2 = Very true or often true**

0 I 2	1.	Acts too young for his/her age
0 I 2	2.	Drinks alcohol without parents' approval (describe): _____ _____
0 I 2	3.	Argues a lot
0 I 2	4.	Fails to finish things he/she starts
0 I 2	5.	There is very little he/she enjoys
0 I 2	6.	Bowel movements outside toilet
0 I 2	7.	Bragging, boasting
0 I 2	8.	Can't concentrate, can't pay attention for long
0 I 2	9.	Can't get his/her mind off certain thoughts; obsessions (describe): _____ _____
0 I 2	10.	Can't sit still, restless, or hyperactive
0 I 2	11.	Clings to adults or too dependent
0 I 2	12.	Complains of loneliness
0 I 2	13.	Confused or seems to be in a fog
0 I 2	14.	Cries a lot
0 I 2	15.	Cruel to animals
0 I 2	16.	Cruelty, bullying, or meanness to others
0 I 2	17.	Daydreams or gets lost in his/her thoughts
0 I 2	18.	Deliberately harms self or attempts suicide
0 I 2	19.	Demands a lot of attention
0 I 2	20.	Destroys his/her own things
0 I 2	21.	Destroys things belonging to his/her family or others
0 I 2	22.	Disobedient at home
0 I 2	23.	Disobedient at school
0 I 2	24.	Doesn't eat well
0 I 2	25.	Doesn't get along with other kids
0 I 2	26	Doesn't seem to feel guilty after misbehaving
0 I 2	27.	Easily jealous
0 I 2	28.	Breaks rules at home, school, or elsewhere
0 I 2	29.	Fears certain animals, situations, or places, other than school (describe): _____ _____
0 I 2	30.	Fears going to school
0 I 2	31.	Fears he/she might think or do something bad

0 I 2	32.	Feels he/she has to be perfect
0 I 2	33.	Feels or complains that no one loves him/her
0 I 2	34.	Feels others are out to get him/her
0 I 2	35.	Feels worthless or inferior
0 I 2	36.	Gets hurt a lot, accident-prone
0 I 2	37.	Gets in many fights
0 I 2	38.	Gets teased a lot
0 I 2	39.	Hangs around with others who get in trouble
0 I 2	40.	Hears sounds or voices that aren't there (describe): _____ _____
0 I 2	41.	Impulsive or acts without thinking
0 I 2	42.	Would rather be alone than with others
0 I 2	43.	Lying or cheating
0 I 2	44.	Bites fingernails
0 I 2	45.	Nervous, highstrung, or tense
0 I 2	46.	Nervous movements or twitching (describe): _____ _____
0 I 2	47.	Nightmares
0 I 2	48.	Not liked by other kids
0 I 2	49.	Constipated, doesn't move bowels
0 I 2	50.	Too fearful or anxious
0 I 2	51.	Feels dizzy or lightheaded
0 I 2	52.	Feels too guilty
0 I 2	53.	Overeating
0 I 2	54.	Overtired without good reason
0 I 2	55.	Overweight
	56.	Physical problems *without known medical cause:*
0 I 2	a.	Aches or pains (*not* stomach or headaches)
0 I 2	b.	Headaches
0 I 2	c.	Nausea, feels sick
0 I 2	d.	Problems with eyes (*not* if corrected by glasses) (describe): _____ _____
0 I 2	e.	Rashes or other skin problems
0 I 2	f.	Stomach aches
0 I 2	g.	Vomiting, throwing up
0 I 2	h.	Other (describe): _____ _____

21

0	I	2	57.	Physically attacks people
0	I	2	58.	Picks nose, skin, or other parts of body (describe):

_____

_____

0	I	2	59.	Plays with own sex parts in public
0	I	2	60.	Plays with own sex parts too much
0	I	2	61.	Poor school work
0	I	2	62.	Poorly coordinated or clumsy
0	I	2	63.	Prefers being with older kids
0	I	2	64.	Prefers being with younger kids
0	I	2	65.	Refuses to talk
0	I	2	66.	Repeats certain acts over and over; compulsions (describe):

_____

0	I	2	67.	Runs away from home
0	I	2	68.	Screams a lot
0	I	2	69.	Secretive, keeps things to self
0	I	2	70.	Sees things that aren't there (describe):

_____

0	I	2	71.	Self-concscious or easily embarrassed
0	I	2	72.	Sets fires
0	I	2	73.	Sexual problems (describe):

_____

0	I	2	74.	Showing off or clowning
0	I	2	75.	Too shy or timid
0	I	2	76.	Sleeps less than most kids
0	I	2	77.	Sleeps more than most kids during day and/or night (describe):

_____

0	I	2	78.	Inattentive or easily distracted
0	I	2	79.	Speech problem (describe):

_____

0	I	2	80.	Stares blankly
0	I	2	81.	Steals at home
0	I	2	83.	Steals outside the home
0	I	2	83.	Stores up too many things he/she doesn't need (describe):

_____

_____

_____

0	I	2	84.	Strange behavior (describe):

_____

0	I	2	85.	Strange ideas (describe):

_____

0	I	2	86.	Stubborn, sullen, or irritable
0	I	2	87.	Sudden changes in mood or feelings
0	I	2	88.	Sulks a lot
0	I	2	89.	Suspicious
0	I	2	90.	Swearing or obscene language
0	I	2	91.	Talks about killing self
0	I	2	92.	Talks or walks in sleep (describe):

_____

0	I	2	93.	Talks too much
0	I	2	94.	Teases a lot
0	I	2	95.	Temper tantrums or hot temper
0	I	2	96.	Thinks about sex too much
0	I	2	97.	Threatens people
0	I	2	98.	Thumb-sucking
0	I	2	99.	Smokes, chews, or sniffs tobacco
0	I	2	100.	Trouble sleeping (describe):

_____

0	I	2	101.	Truancy, skips school
0	I	2	102.	Underactive, slow moving, or lacks energy
0	I	2	103.	Unhappy, sad, or depressed
0	I	2	104.	Unusually loud
0	I	2	105.	Uses drugs for nonmedical purposes (**don't** include alcohol or tobacco) (describe):

_____

0	I	2	106.	Vandalism
0	I	2	107.	Wets self during the day
0	I	2	108.	Wets the bed
0	I	2	109.	Whining
0	I	2	110.	Wishes to be of opposite sex
0	I	2	111.	Withdrawn, doesn't get involved with others
0	I	2	112.	Worries
			113.	Please write in any problems your child has that were not listed above:
0	I	2		_____
0	I	2		_____
0	I	2		_____

Please be sure you answered all items

Behavior Assessment System for Children – Second Edition (BASC-2)

Time PRS: 10–20 minutes. TRS: 10–15 minutes. SRP: 20–30 minutes

Ages PRS: 2–5, 6–11, 12–21; TRS: 2–5, 6–11, 12–21; SRP: 8–11, 12–21

Time Frame PRS, TRS: last several months; SRP: not specified

Purpose Assessment of emotional and behavioral problems, adaptive functioning and personality.

Commentary

The BASC-2 was published in 2004 and is the successor of the BASC that was conceptualized in 1985 and published in 1992.

Versions

The Behavior Assessment System for Children – Second Edition (BASC-2) comprises Parent Rating Scales (PRS), Teacher Rating Scales (TRS), and the Self-Report of Personality (SRP). Each type of rating scale includes forms for three age levels. Recently, a fourth level for the SRP was released. The SRP-Interview was designed for 6 and 7 year olds. Its items are read to the child. In addition, the BASC-2 comprises a Structured Developmental History (SDH) form and a Student Observation System (SOS) for recording and classifying directly observed classroom behavior, but these will not be described here.

Properties

Items The PRS contains 134–160 and the TRS 100–139 items concerning emotional and behavioral problems and adaptive behavior. All items of the PRS and TRS are rated on a 4-point scale, with responses: never, sometimes, often, and almost always. The SRP contains 139–185 items on emotions and self-perceptions. Most items of the SRP are also rated on the same 4-point scale, but the rest of the items are scored on a true-false scale.

Scales The PRS, TRS, and SRP can be scored on three types of scales: primary scales, composite scales, and content scales.

The primary scales are based on factor analysis of the items. The common primary scales of the PRS and TRS

are Adaptability, Aggression, Anxiety, Attention Problems, Atypicality, Conduct Problems, Depression, Functional Communication, Hyperactivity, Leadership, Social Skills, Somatization, Withdrawal. In addition, the PRS includes Activities of Daily Living, and the TRS includes Learning Problems and Study Skills. The primary scales of the SRP are Anxiety, Attention Problems, Attitude to School, Attitude to teachers, Atypicality, Depression, Hyperactivity, Interpersonal relations, Locus of Control, Relations with parents, Self-Esteem, Self-Reliance, Sensation Seeking, Sense of Inadequacy, Social Stress, Somatization.

Composite scales are based on factor analysis of the primary scales. The composite scales of both the PRS and TRS are Adaptive Skills, Behavioral Symptoms Index, Externalizing Problems, Internalizing Problems. In addition, the TRS includes School Problems. The composite scales of the SRP are Emotional Symptoms Index, Inattention/Hyperactivity, Internalizing Problems, Personal Adjustment, School Problems.

Content scales consist of a combination of both items belonging to the primary scales and items not a part of any primary scale. The content scales of both the PRS and TRS are Anger Control, Bullying, Developmental Social Disorders, Emotional Self-Control, Executive Functioning, Negative Emotionality, Resiliency. The content scales of the SRP are Anger Control, Ego Strength, Mania, Test Anxiety.

In addition, the PRS, TRS, SRP comprise validity indexes for assessing the quality of a completed form. The F index on the PRS, TRS, and SRP indicates the respondent's tendency to be excessively negative, The L index on the SRP indicates the child's tendency to be extremely positive, the V Index on the SRP indicates the validity of the SRP scores in general. The Consistency Index and the Response Pattern Index on the PRS, TRS, and SRP are available in the computer program. They detect whether respondents disregard item content and give inconsistent or patterned responses.

Reliability Median test-retest correlations over 8 to 70-days intervals ranged from 0.76 to 0.84 for the PRS, from 0.79 to 0.88 for the TRS, and from 0.71 to 0.84 for the SRP.

Median Cronbach's alphas across scales per age and norm group ranged from 0.80 to 0.87 for the PRS, from 0.84 to 0.89 for the TRS, and from 0.75 to 0.86 for the SRP.

Validity Correlations of BASC-2 scales with scales that measure similar constructs were generally high, although correlations for internalizing scales across instruments were more variable than for externalizing scales.

Norms The BASC-2 was standardized on 4800 PRS ratings, 4650 TRS ratings, and 3400 SRP ratings from the general population and on 1975 PRS ratings, 1779 TRS ratings, and 1527 ratings from clinical samples. Raw scores were converted to T-scores and percentiles.

Use Supplementary materials include a manual describing all BASC-2 forms, hand-scoring profiles, a computer program for data entry and scoring.

Key references

Reynolds CR, Kamphaus RW. Behavior Assessment System for Children – Second Edition: Manual. Circle Pines, MN: AGS Publishing, 2004.

Address

AGS Publishing
4201 Woodland Road
Circle Pines, MN 55014–1796
USA
www.agsnet.com

Brief Psychiatric Rating Scale for Children (BPRS-C)

Time 5 minutes

Ages 5–18

Time Frame Not specified

Purpose Assessment of emotional and behavioral problems.

Commentary

The BPRS-C was developed to assess variations in problems among child and adolescent patients, and to assess changes in problem scores to various treatments through repeated administering (Overall and Pfefferbaum, 1982). It focuses on problems as scored by clinicians, and thereby complements clinician ratings of functional impairment. Extensions of the original BPRS-C appeared in which descriptive anchors were added to items to improve reliability and validity for trained and untrained raters (for example Hughes et al, 2001). The BPRS-C has been widely used in research to quantify the effects of medication.

Versions

The Brief Psychiatric Rating Scale for Children (BPRS-C) is only available as a clinician-rated scale.

Properties

Items The BPRS-C comprises 21 items that are rated on a 7-point scale with responses: not present, very mild, mild, moderate, moderately severe, severe, and extremely severe.

Scales Factor analysis supported 7 subscales, each consisting of 3 items. The subscales are labeled: Behavior Problems, Depression, Thinking Disturbance, Psychomotor Excitation, Withdrawal-Retardation, Anxiety, and Organicity. Although a total score was not originally described, it is often used as an indication of overall severity.

Reliability Interrater reliability of item ratings of 48 patients by three raters ranged from 0.46 to 0.89.

Cronbach's alphas ranged from 0.69 to 0.91 for the 7 subscales of the BPRS-C in a sample of 48 patients.

Validity

The Anxiety and Depression subscales correlated 0.35 and 0.28, respectively with self-reported anxiety, and 0.27 and 0.19, respectively with self-reported depression in a group of child psychiatric patients.

Norms No information available.

Use The BPRS-C is published in Overall and Pfefferbaum (1982).

Key references

Gale J, Pfefferbaum, Suhr MA, Overall JE. The Brief Psychiatric Rating Scale for Children: A reliability study. J Clin Child Psychol 1986; 15: 341–5.

Hughes CW, Rintelmann J, Emslie GJ, Lopez M, MacCabe N. A revised anchored version of the BPRS-C for childhood psychiatric disorders. J Child Adolesc Psychopharmacol 2001; 11: 77–93.

Overall JE, Pfefferbaum B. The Brief Psychiatric Rating Scale for Children. Psychopharmacol Bull 1982; 18: 10–16.

Address

John E. Overall
Department of Psychiatry and Behavioral Science
The University of Texas Health Science Center at Houston
7000 Fannin, Suite 1200
Houston, Texas 77030
USA
john.e.overall@uth.tmc.edu

Child Symptom Inventories (CSI)

Time 15–20 minutes

Ages ECI-4: 3–5; CSI-4: 5–12; ASI-4: 12–18; YI: 12–18

Time Frame Not specified

Purpose Assessment of emotional and behavioral problems.

Commentary

The development of the CSI started in 1984 with a rating scale that was based on the DSM. The first version only assessed a few problem areas, but was subsequently extended to cover more problem areas and that could be completed by multiple informants for children across a wide age range. The current CSI-4 are based on the DSM-IV criteria and cover over a dozen disorders.

Versions

The Child Symptom Inventories (CSI) are available in several forms for different age groups and informants. The Early Childhood Inventory-4 (ECI-4) is available as parent and teacher reports for ages 3–5 years (preschool). The Child Symptom Inventory-4 (CSI-4) is available as parent and teacher reports for ages 5–12 years (elementary school). The Adolescent Symptom Inventory-4 (ASI-4) is available as a parent and teacher report and the Youth's Inventory-4 (YI-4) is available as a self-report for ages 12–18 years (secondary school).

Properties

Items Depending on age group and informant, the CSI comprise 77 to 120 items. Most items are rated on a 4-point scale with responses: never, sometimes, often, and very often. The rest of the items are rated on a 2-point scale with responses: yes, and no.

Scales The items of the CSI are scored on subscales in two different ways. First, for Symptom Count scores, items are first dichotomized (generally, never = 0; sometimes = 0; often = 1; very often = 1) and the item counts for each subscale are then compared to criterion scores based on DSM-IV criteria. When an item count is

greater than or equal to a criterion score, the Screening Cutoff is set to yes, and when an item count is lower than a criterion score, the Screening Cutoff is set to no.

Second, the Symptom Severity scores are computed by summing item scores per subscale. The yes-no rated items are assigned weights to make them comparable to items rated on a 4-point scale (never = 0; very often = 3; no = 0.5; yes = 2.5).

For both scoring methods, subscale scores represent disorders as defined by the DSM-IV. The following disorders are covered by the CSI, although variations exist across age groups and informants: AD/HD; Oppositional Defiant Disorder; Conduct Disorder; Generalized Anxiety Disorder; Social Phobia; Separation Anxiety Disorder; Obsessive-Compulsive Disorder; Specific Phobia; Panic Attacks; Selective Mutism; Major Depressive Disorder; Dysthymic Disorder; Bipolar Disorder; Reactive Attachment Disorder; Schizophrenia; Pervasive Developmental Disorder; Asperger's Disorder; Motor Tics; Vocal Tics; Posttraumatic Stress Disorder; Problems in Eating, Sleeping, Elimination; Bulimia; Anorexia Nervosa; Somatization Disorder; Antisocial Personality Disorder; Schizoid Personality Disorder; Drug Use. Depending on age group and informant, 13–18 disorders are scored. The composition of subscales was partially supported by factor analysis.

In addition to the DSM-IV based subscales, the ECI-4 also includes the Peer Conflict Scale assessing interpersonal peer aggression and the Developmental Deficits Index assessing for language, motor, and self-help skills, play behaviors, and responsiveness to adults.

Reliability Test–retest correlations for the Symptom Severity scores ranged 0.35–0.85 across a 3-month interval for the parent ECI-4 in school children, 0.62–0.90 across a 2-day interval of ADHD and ODD ratings, except a correlation of 0.38 for ADHD Hyperactive-Impulsive, for the teacher ECI-4 in a clinical trial, 0.46–0.87 across a 4-week interval for the parent CSI-4 in clinical children, 0.68–0.88 across a 2-week interval for the teacher CSI-4 in a special education sample, 0.54–0.92 across a 2-week interval for the YI-4 in a special education sample.

Cronbach's alphas for Symptom Severity scores ranged 0.59–0.93 for the parent and 0.66–0.95 for the teacher ECI-4, 0.74–0.94 for the parent and 0.70–0.96 for the teacher CSI-4, 0.61–0.95 for the parent, and 0.71–0.97 for the teacher ASI-4, and 0.66–0.87 for the self-report YI-4.

Validity Correlations of the Symptom Severity scores with corresponding scales of other general rating scales for emotional and behavioral problems ranged from 0.30 to 0.81 for the parent ECI-4, from 0.31 to 0.87 for the teacher ECI-4, from 0.47 to 0.70 for the parent CSI-4, from 0.58 to 0.82 for the teacher CSI-4, from 0.51 to 0.80 for the parent ASI-4, from 0.52 to 0.90 for the teacher ASI-4, and from 0.48 to 0.74 for the self-report YI-4.

Screening Cutoff scores of the CSI were compared with child psychiatrists' diagnoses in samples of clinical children. The Screening Cutoff scores distinguished between children with and without diagnoses for several disorders with sensitivities and specificities ranging 72–74% and 54–74%, respectively for the parent ECI-4, 54–89% and 75–100%, respectively for the teacher ECI-4, 38–100% and 63–99%, respectively for the parent CSI-4, 38–89% and 62–99%, respectively for the teacher CSI-4, 50–100% and 53–100%, respectively for the parent ASI-4, 10–71% and 64–99%, respectively for the teacher ASI-4, and 31–75% and 78–98%, respectively for the self-report YI-4.

Mean Symptom Severity scores were significantly higher for clinical children than for children in the normative samples. This was true for the parent ECI-4, except the scores of girls for Separation Anxiety Disorder, for the parent CSI-4, except the scores of boys for Separation Anxiety Disorder, and for the teacher CSI-4. However, for the YI-4 only a few differences were significant. For males, differences were significant for ADHD Inattentive, ADHD Combined, Oppositional Defiant Disorder, Conduct Disorder, and Schizoid Personality. For females, differences were significant for ADHD Inattentive and Vocal Tics.

Norms For the standardization of the CSI children were recruited through pediatricians, day care centers, preschools, and elementary, middle, and high schools in the USA. The CSI were standardized on 531 parent ratings and 398 teacher ratings for the ECI-4, on 551 parent ratings and 1323 teacher ratings for the CSI-4, on 761 parent ratings and 1072 teacher ratings for the ASI-4, and on 573 self-report ratings for the YI-4. Raw scores are converted to T-scores and percentile scores.

Use Manuals, rating scales, scoring profiles, and a computer program for scoring and reporting can be obtained from the publisher at the address below.

Key references

Gadow KD, Sprafkin J. Adolescent Symptom Inventory-4 Screening manual. Stony Brook, NY: Checkmate Plus, LTD, 1997.

Gadow KD, Sprafkin J. Early Childhood Inventory-4 Norms manual. Stony Brook, NY: Checkmate Plus, LTD, 1997.

Gadow KD, Sprafkin J. Adolescent Symptom Inventory-4 Norms manual. Stony Brook, NY: Checkmate Plus, Ltd, 1998.

Gadow KD, Sprafkin J. Youth's Inventory-4 manual. Stony Brook, NY: Checkmate Plus, Ltd, 1999.

Gadow KD, Sprafkin J. Early Childhood Inventory-4 Screening manual. Stony Brook, NY: Checkmate Plus, Ltd, 2000.

Gadow KD, Sprafkin J. Child Symptom Inventory-4 Screening and Norms manual. Stony Brook, NY: Checkmate Plus, Ltd, 2002.

Gadow KD, Sprafkin J, Carlson GA, et al. A DSM-IV-referenced, adolescent self-report rating scale. J Am Acad Child Adolesc Psychiatry 2002; 41: 671–9.

Gadow KD, Sprafkin J, Salisbury H, Schnieder J, Coney J. Futher validity evidence for the teacher version of the Child Symptom Inventory-4. School Psychology Quarterly 2004; 19: 50–71.

Mattison RE, Gadow KD, Sprafkin J, Nolan EE, Schneider J. A DSM-IV-referred teacher rating scale for use in clinical management. J Am Acad Child Adolesc Psychiatry 2003; 42: 444–9.

Sprafkin J, Gadow KD, Schneider J, Coney J. Further evidence of reliability and validity of the Child Symptom Inventory-4: parent checklist in clinically referred boys. J Clin Child Adolesc Psychol. 2002; 31: 513–24.

Sprafkin J, Volpe RJ, Gadow KD, Nolan EN, Kelly K. A DSM-IV-referenced screening instrument for preschool children: The Early Childhood Inventory-4. J Am Acad Child Adolesc Psychiatry 2002; 41: 604–12.

Address

Checkmate Plus
PO Box 696
Stony Brook, NY 11790–0696
USA
www.checkmateplus.com

Child Symptom Inventory-4 (CSI-4) – Parent checklist – sample page

Category B	Never	Sometimes	Often	Very often
19. Loses temper	❑	❑	❑	❑
20. Argues with adults	❑	❑	❑	❑
21. Defies or refuses what you tell him/her to do	❑	❑	❑	❑
22. Does things to deliberately annoy others	❑	❑	❑	❑
23. Blames others for own misbehavior or mistakes	❑	❑	❑	❑
24. Is touchy or easily annoyed by others	❑	❑	❑	❑
25. Is angry and resentful	❑	❑	❑	❑
26. Takes anger out on others or tries to get even	❑	❑	❑	❑

Category C	Never	Sometimes	Often	Very often
27. Plays hookey from school	❑	❑	❑	❑
28. Stays out at night when not supposed to	❑	❑	❑	❑
29. Lies to get things or to avoid responsibility ('cons' others)	❑	❑	❑	❑
30. Bullies, threatens, or intimidates others	❑	❑	❑	❑
31. Starts physical fights	❑	❑	❑	❑
32. Has run away from home overnight	❑	❑	❑	❑
33. Has stolen things when others were not looking	❑	❑	❑	❑
34. Has deliberately destroyed others' property	❑	❑	❑	❑
35. Has deliberately started fires	❑	❑	❑	❑
36. Has stolen things from others using physical force	❑	❑	❑	❑
37. Has broken into someone else's house, building, or car	❑	❑	❑	❑
38. Has used a weapon when fighting (bat, brick, bottle, etc.)	❑	❑	❑	❑
39. Has been physically cruel to animals	❑	❑	❑	❑
40. Has been physically cruel to people	❑	❑	❑	❑
41. Has been preoccupied with or involved in sexual activity	❑	❑	❑	❑

Category D	Never	Sometimes	Often	Very often
42. Is overconcerned about abilities in academic, athletic, or social activities	❑	❑	❑	❑
43. Has difficulty controlling worries	❑	❑	❑	❑
44. Acts restless or edgy	❑	❑	❑	❑
45. Is irritable for most of the day	❑	❑	❑	❑
46. Is extremely tense or unable to relax	❑	❑	❑	❑
47. Has difficulty falling asleep or staying asleep	❑	❑	❑	❑
48. Complains about physical problems (headaches, upset stomach, etc.) for which there is no apparent cause	❑	❑	❑	❑

Conners' Rating Scales – Revised (CRS-R)

Time 15–20 minutes

Ages CPRS-R: 3–17; CTRS-R: 3–17; CASS: 12–17

Time Frame CPRS-R: Last month; CTRS-R: Last month; CASS: No time frame given

Purpose Assessment of emotional and behavioral problems.

Commentary

Development of the CRS started more than forty years ago and resulted in official publication in 1989. In 1997 the parent and teacher forms were revised and a new self-report form was added. Over 11 000 cases were collected to test the new CRS-R forms.

Versions

The Conners' Rating Scales-Revised (CRS-R) comprise the Conners' Parent Rating Scale-Revised (CPRS-R), the Conners' Teacher Rating Scale-Revised (CTRS-R), and the Conners-Wells' Adolescent Self-Report Scale (CASS). For each rating scale, long versions as well as short versions exist. Several items from the long versions are taken to form Conners' ADHD/DSM-IV Scales (CADS).

Properties

Items The CPRS-R has 80 items, the CTRS-R 59, and the CASS 87. The corresponding short versions have 27, 28, and 27 items, respectively. All items are scored on a 4-point scale with responses: not true at all, just a little true, pretty much true, very much true.

Scales All three versions comprise subscales derived from exploratory and confirmative factor analyses. The CPRS-R comprises 7 subscales: Oppositional, Cognitive Problems/Inattention, Hyperactivity, Anxious-Shy, Perfectionism, Social Problems, and Psychosomatic. The CTRS-R comprises the same subscales, except Psychosomatic. The CASS comprises 6 subscales: Family Problems, Emotional Problems, Conduct Problems, Cognitive Problems/Inattention, Anger Control, and Hyperactivity.

All three versions also comprise two subscales with ADHD symptoms. The DSM-IV Symptoms subscale corresponds with symptoms used in the DSM and can be further divided into two subscales called Inattentive and Hyperactive-Impulsive. The ADHD Index comprises items that identify ADHD children.

Both CPRS-R and CTRS-R contain the subscale Conners' Global Index that can be further divided into two subscales called Restless-Impulsive and Emotional Lability.

Reliability Test–retest correlations over a 6–8-week interval ranged from 0.47 to 0.85 for the CPRS-R, from 0.47 to 0.88 for the CTRS-R, and 0.73 to 0.89 for the CASS.

Cronbach's alphas ranged from 0.73 to 0.94 for the CPRS-R, from 0.77 to 0.96 for the CTRS-R, and from 0.74 to 0.94 for the CASS.

Validity Moderate to high correlations were found between most of the scales of the CPRS-R, CTRS-R, and the CASS and a self-report measure of depression. The CPRS-R DSM-IV Symptoms Inattentive subscale correlated significantly with an attention performance test, while other hyperactivity and inattention subscales correlated non-significantly.

The DSM-IV Symptoms subscales of the CPRS-L and CTRS-R were used to identify children and adolescents who were meeting diagnostic criteria for ADHD. The ADHD group had significantly higher scores on all scales of the CPRS-R and CTRS-R than the non-ADHD group, with the exception of the Perfectionism scale. The scales of the CPRS-R, CTRS-R, and CASS discriminated well among three groups of children and adolescents who were diagnosed as having ADHD, were not having problems, and were rated as having emotional problems.

Norms The CRS-R were standardized on 2482 CPRS-R ratings, 1973 CTRS-R ratings, and 3394 CASS ratings of children and adolescents from the general population. For interpretation of the CRS-R raw scores were converted to percentiles and T-scores.

Use Supplementary materials include a manual describing all CRS-R forms, scoring profiles, a computer program for data entry and scoring and are available from the publisher at the address below.

Key references

Conners CK. Conners' Rating Scales – Revised. North Tonawanda, NY: Multi-Health Systems Inc, 1997.

Conners CK, Sitarenios G, Parker JDA, Epstein. The revised Conners' Parent Rating Scale (CPRS-R): Factor structure, reliability, and criterion validity. J Abnorm Child Psychol 1998; 26: 257–68.

Conners CK, Sitarenios G, Parker JDA, Epstein. Revision and restandardization of the Conners' Teacher Rating Scale (CTRS-R): Factor structure, reliability, and criterion validity. J Abnorm Child Psychol 1998; 26: 279–91.

Conners CK, Wells KC, Parker JDA, et al. A new self-report scale for the assessment of adolescent psychopathology: Factor structure, reliability, validity, and diagnostic sensitivity. J Abnorm Child Psychol 1997; 25: 487–97.

Address

Multi-Health Systems Inc.
P.O. Box 950
North Tonawanda, NY 14120–0950
USA
www.mhs.com

Conners' Rating Scales – Revised (CRS-R) – sample items

Conners' Parent Rating Scale-Revised (L)

	Not true at all (Never, seldom)	Just a little true (Occasionally)	Pretty much true (Often, quite a bit)	Very much true (Very often, very frequent)
11. Argues with adults	0	1	2	3
12. Fails to complete assignments	0	1	2	3
13. Hard to control in malls or while grocery shopping	0	1	2	3
14. Afraid of people	0	1	2	3
15. Keeps checking things over again and again	0	1	2	3
16. Loses friends quickly	0	1	2	3

Conners' Teacher Rating Scale-Revised (L)

	Not true at all (Never, seldom)	Just a little true (Occasionally)	Pretty much true (Often, quite a bit)	Very much true (Very often, very frequent)
28. Has difficulty sustaining attention in tasks or play activities	0	1	2	3
29. Has difficulty waiting his/her turn	0	1	2	3
30. Not reading up to par	0	1	2	3
31. Does not know how to make friends	0	1	2	3
32. Sensitive to criticism	0	1	2	3
33. Seems over-focused on details	0	1	2	3

Conners-Wells' Adolescent Self-Report Scale (L)

	Not true at all (Never, seldom)	Just a little true (Occasionally)	Pretty much true (Often, quite a bit)	Very much true (Very often, very frequent)
68. Sometimes I feel like I am driven by a motor	0	1	2	3
69. I am touchy or easily annoyed	0	1	2	3
70. I am always on the go	0	1	2	3
71. My parents do not really care about me	0	1	2	3
72. The future seems hopeless to me	0	1	2	3
73. I take things that do not belong to me	0	1	2	3

Devereux Scales of Mental Disorders (DSMD)

Time 20 minutes

Ages 5–18

Time Frame Last 4 weeks

Purpose Assessment of emotional and behavioral problems.

Commentary

The DSMD are revisions of rating scales that first appeared in 1964 (Spivack and Levine, 1964). The goal in developing the DSMD was to formalize the assessment of a large and representative set of behaviors associated with psychopathology.

Versions

The Devereux Scales of Mental Disorders (DSMD) comprise separate forms for ages 5–12 and 13–18 years. Both forms can be completed by parents or teachers.

Properties

Items   The DSMD comprise 111 items for ages 5–12 and 110 items for ages 13–18 that are rated on a 5-point scale with responses: never, rarely, occasionally, frequently, and very frequently.

Scales   The items can be scored on 6 subscales for each age group, which are supported by factor analysis. The subscales are: Conduct, Attention (only for ages 5–12), Delinquency (only for ages 13–18), Anxiety, Depression, Autism, and Acute Problems. These subscales can be combined into Composites: Externalizing, consisting of Conduct and Attention for ages 5–12 and of Conduct and Delinquency for ages 13–18; Internalizing consisting of Anxiety and Depression; and Critical Pathology consisting of Autism and Acute Problems. In addition, the Total Scale is the simple sum of all item ratings.

Reliability   Test–retest correlations across a 24-hour interval ranged from 0.75 to 0.95 for subscales and from 0.85 to 0.91 for Composites and the Total Scale for teacher ratings and ranged from 0.41 to 0.79 for subscales and from 0.49 to 0.85 for Composites and the Total Scale for staff ratings in a clinical sample. Test–retest correlations corrected for restriction of range across a 1-week interval ranged from 0.61 to 0.97 for subscales and from 0.79 to 0.96 for Composites and the Total Scale for

teacher ratings in a sample of school children.

Cronbach's alphas ranged from 0.70 to 0.99 for the subscales, from 0.88 to 0.98 for Composites, and from 0.97 to 0.98 for the Total Scale across rater, gender, and age in the standardization sample.

Validity   Mean T-scores were highest for Conduct and Delinquency in a sample of children with conduct disorder; for Conduct and Attention in a sample of children with ADHD; for Depression in a sample of children with depressive disorder; for Autism in a sample of children with autistic disorder; for Depression, Autism, and Acute Problems in a sample of children with psychotic disorder. A sample of children with anxiety disorder had elevated T-scores on all subscales.

Children in psychiatric hospitals, children in residential treatment centers, children with emotional and learning problems in schools, and children in special education programs for serious emotional problems had significantly higher subscale, Composites, and Total Scale T-scores than matched control children. Accuracy rates in these comparisons for identifying children with psychopathology ranged from 70% to 90%.

Norms   The DSMD was standardized on 3153 parent and teacher ratings of children aged 5–18 years from the US general population. Raw scores were converted into T-scores and percentile ranks.

Use   A manual and rating scaling enabling direct scoring are available from the publisher at the address below.

Key references

Naglieri JA, LeBuffe PA, Pfeiffer SI. Devereux Scales of Mental Disorders Manual. San Antonio: The Psychological Corporation, 1994.

Spivack G, Levine M. The Devereux Child Behavior rating scales: A study of symptom behaviors in latency age atypical children. Am J Ment Defic 1964; 68: 700–17.

Address

Harcourt Assessment
Procter House
1 Procter Street
London WC1V 6EU
United Kingdom
www.harcourt-uk.com

Pediatric Symptom Checklist (PSC)

Time 5 minutes

Ages 4–16

Time Frame Not specified

Purpose Assessment of emotional and behavioral problems.

Commentary

The PSC was developed to facilitate recognition and referral of psychosocial problems as part of routine primary care visits. Therefore, it was designed as a short parent-reported questionnaire. Recent extensions of the PSC are a self-report and a teacher report, and scoring of items on subscales.

Versions

The Pediatric Symptom Checklist (PSC) comprises a parent and a self-report form.

Properties

Items The PSC comprises 35 items that are rated on a 3-point scale with responses: never, sometimes, and often.

Scales The items are scored on a total score which is the simple sum of all item ratings.

Reliability Test–retest correlations across 4-week intervals for parent reports were 0.86 and 0.84 in pediatric outpatient samples.

Cronbach's alpha was 0.89 for parent reports in a pediatric outpatient sample and 0.91 for parent reports of children who visited health clinics.

Validity The PSC cut-off score of 28 has a sensitivity of 95% and a specificity of 68% when compared to clinicians' ratings of children's dysfunction.

Norms No information available.

Use Information about the PSC is given on the website psc.partners.org, where rating scales can be downloaded as well.

Key references

Jellinek M, Evans N, Knight RB. Use of a behavior checklist on a pediatric inpatient unit. J Pediatr 1979 ; 94: 156–8.

Jellinek MS, Murphy JM. Screening for psychosocial disorders in pediatric practice. Am J Dis Child 1988; 142: 1153–7.

Jellinek MS, Murphy JM, Robinson J, et al. Pediatric Symptom Checklist: Screening school-age children for psychosocial dysfunction. J Pediatr 1988; 112: 201–9.

Murphy JM, Ichinose C, Hicks RC, et al. Utility of the Pediatric Symptom Checklist as a psychosocial screen to meet the federal Early and Periodic Screening, Diagnosis, and Treatment (EPSDT) standards: A pilot study. J Pediatr 1996; 129: 864–9.

Murphy JM, Reede J, Jellinek MS, Bishop SJ. Screening for psychosocial dysfunction in inner-city children: Further validation of the Pediatric Symptom Checklist. J Am Acad Child Adolesc Psychiatry 1992; 31: 1105–11.

Address

Michael S. Jellinek
Michael M. Murphy
Child Psychiatry
Bulfinch 351
Massachusetts General Hospital
Boston, MA 02114
USA
mmurphy6@partners.org
psc.partners.org

Pediatric Symptom Checklist (PSC)

Emotional and physical health go together in children. Because parents are often the first to notice a problem with their child's behavior, emotions or learning, you may help your child get the best care possible by answering these questions. Please indicate which statement best describes your child.

Please mark under the heading that best describes your child:		Never	Sometimes	Often
1. Complains of aches and pains	1	_____	_____	_____
2. Spends more time alone	2	_____	_____	_____
3. Tires easily, has little energy	3	_____	_____	_____
4. Fidgety, unable to sit still	4	_____	_____	_____
5. Has trouble with teacher	5	_____	_____	_____
6. Less interested in school	6	_____	_____	_____
7. Acts as if driven by a motor	7	_____	_____	_____
8. Daydreams too much	8	_____	_____	_____
9. Distracted easily	9	_____	_____	_____
10. Is afraid of new situations	10	_____	_____	_____
11. Feels sad, unhappy	11	_____	_____	_____
12. Is irritable, angry	12	_____	_____	_____
13. Feels hopeless	13	_____	_____	_____
14. Has trouble concentrating	14	_____	_____	_____
15. Less interested in friends	15	_____	_____	_____
16. Fights with other children	16	_____	_____	_____
17. Absent from school	17	_____	_____	_____
18. School grades dropping	18	_____	_____	_____
19. Is down on him or herself	19	_____	_____	_____
20. Visits the doctor with doctor finding nothing wrong	20	_____	_____	_____
21. Has trouble sleeping	21	_____	_____	_____
22. Worries a lot	22	_____	_____	_____
23. Wants to be with you more than before	23	_____	_____	_____
24. Feels he or she is bad	24	_____	_____	_____
25. Takes unnecessary risks	25	_____	_____	_____
26. Gets hurt frequently	26	_____	_____	_____
27. Seems to be having less fun	27	_____	_____	_____
28. Acts younger than children his or her age	28	_____	_____	_____
29. Does not listen to rules	29	_____	_____	_____
30. Does not show feelings	30	_____	_____	_____
31. Does not understand other people's feelings	31	_____	_____	_____
32. Teases others	32	_____	_____	_____
33. Blames others for his or her troubles	33	_____	_____	_____
34. Takes things that do not belong to him or her	34	_____	_____	_____
35. Refuses to share	35	_____	_____	_____

Total score _____

Does your child have any emotional or behavioral problems for which she/he needs help?   ( ) N   ( ) Y

Are there any services that you would like your child to receive for these problems?   ( ) N   ( ) N

If yes, what services? _____

Pediatric Symptom Checklist – Youth Report (Y-PSC)

Please mark under the heading that bests fit you:	Never	Sometimes	Often
1. Complains of aches and pains			
2. Spends more time alone			
3. Tires easily, has little energy			
4. Fidgety, unable to sit still			
5. Has trouble with teacher			
6. Less interested in school			
7. Acts as if driven by a motor			
8. Daydreams too much			
9. Distracted easily			
10. Is afraid of new situations			
11. Feels sad, unhappy			
12. Is irritable, angry			
13. Feels hopeless			
14. Has trouble concentrating			
15. Less interested in friends			
16. Fights with other children			
17. Absent from school			
18. School grades dropping			
19. Is down on him or herself			
20. Visits the doctor with doctor finding nothing wrong			
21. Has trouble sleeping			
22. Worries a lot			
23. Wants to be with you more than before			
24. Feels he or she is bad			
25. Takes unnecessary risks			
26. Gets hurt frequently			
27. Seems to be having less fun			
28. Acts younger than children his or her age			
29. Does not listen to rules			
30. Does not show feelings			
31. Does not understand other people's feelings			
32. Teases others			
33. Blames others for his or her troubles			
34. Takes things that do not belong to him or her			
35. Refuses to share			

Revised Behavior Problem Checklist (RBPC)

Time 15 minutes

Ages 5–18

Time Frame Not specified

Purpose Assessment of emotional and behavioral problems.

Commentary

The RBPC is a revision of the Behavior Problem Checklist that appeared in 1977.

Versions

The Revised Behavior Problem Checklist (RBPC) comprises only one version to be completed by parents or teachers.

Properties

Items   The RBPC comprises 89 items that are rated on a 3-point scale with responses: not a problem, mild problem, and severe problem.

Scales   The items of the RBPC are scored on 6 scales derived from factor analyses in clinical samples, which are labeled Conduct Disorder, Socialized Aggression, Attention Problems-Immaturity, Anxiety-Withdrawal, Psychotic Behavior, Motor Tension-Excess.

Reliability   Test–retest correlations across a 2-month interval ranged from 0.49 to 0.83.
    Cronbach's alphas ranged from 0.68 to 0.95.

Validity   Correlations with behavioral observations, peer nominations and other rating scales demonstrated convergent and discriminant validity.
    Both teacher and parent ratings of all scales were significantly different between normal and clinical children.

Norms   The teacher ratings of the RBPC were standardized on 972 unselected public school children and 270 emotionally disturbed children. Raw scores were converted to normalized T-scores. In addition, the manual provides tables with means and standard deviations of both teacher and parent ratings for normal and clinical samples.

Use   A manual and rating scales enabling direct scoring are available from the publisher at the address below.

Key references

Quay HC, Peterson DR. RBPC Revised Behavior Problem Checklist: Professional Manual. Lutz, Fl: Psychological Assessment Resources, Inc, 1996.

Address

Psychological Assessment Resources, Inc.
16204 N. Florida Avenue
Lutz, FL 33549
USA
www.parinc.com

Revised Behavior Problem Checklist (RBPC) – sample items

	Not a problem	Mild problem	Severe problem
32. Destructive in regard to own and/or other's properties	0	1	2
77. Cannot stand to wait; wants everything now	0	1	2

Strengths and Difficulties Questionnaire (SDQ)

Time 5 minutes

Ages 4–16

Time Frame Last 6 months

Purpose Assessment of emotional and behavioral problems and prosocial behavior.

Commentary

The SDQ is an adaptation of the Rutter's scales and is translated into more than 50 languages.

Versions

The Strengths and Difficulties Questionnaire (SDQ) comprises forms to be completed by parents, teachers or youths from 11 years themselves.

Properties

Items The SDQ comprises 25 problem items that are rated on a 3-point scale with responses: not true, somewhat true, and certainly true. In addition, the SDQ can be extended with a brief impact supplement that comprises 8 items on the parent and self-report forms and 6 items on the teacher form rated on a 4-point scale.

Scales Factor analysis supported 5 factors, therefore, the problem items of the SDQ are scored on 5 scales, which are labeled Emotional Symptoms, Conduct Problems, Hyperactivity-Inattention, Peer Problems, Prosocial Behavior. In addition, the sum of all items, except the items of the Prosocial Behavior scale constitutes the Total Difficulties scale. The items on overall distress and social impairment of the impact supplement can be scored on the Impact scale.

Reliability Test–retest correlations across a 4–6-month interval ranged from 0.21 to 0.82.
 Cronbach's alphas ranged from 0.41 to 0.88.

Validity Odds ratios from the comparison of SDQ scales with conceptually similar DSM-IV diagnoses were higher than odds ratios from the comparison with conceptually different diagnoses.

Norms The SDQ was standardized on 10 298 parent ratings, 8208 teacher ratings, and 4224 self-reports of children from the British general population.

Use Tables with means and standard deviations and with frequency distributions of ratings of children from the British general population and of ratings from the American general population are available from the website, where also references can be found for normative data from Finland, Germany and Sweden. In addition, the website has forms available for download for more than 50 languages.

Key references

Bourdon, Goodman R, Rae DS, Simpson G, Koretz D. The Strengths and Difficulties Questionnaire: U.S. normative date and psychometric properties. J Am Acad Child Adolesc Psychiatry 2001; 44: 557–64.

Goodman R. The Strengths and Difficulties Questionnaire: A research note. J Child Psychol Psychiatry 1997; 38: 581–6.

Goodman R. Psychometric properties of the Strengths and Difficulties Questionnaire. J Am Acad Child Adolesc Psychiatry 2001; 40: 1337–45.

Goodman R, Meltzer H, Bailey V. The Strengths and Difficulties Questionnaire: a pilot study on the validity of the self-report version. Eur Child Adolesc Psychiatry 1998; 7: 125–30.

Address

Robert Goodman
Box PO85
Department of Child and Adolescent Psychiatry
Institute of Psychiatry
King's College London
London SE5 8AF
UK
r.goodman@iop.kcl.ac.uk
www.sdqinfo.com

Chapter 3

Scales for Specific Problems

3.1 Anxiety

Affect and Arousal Scale (AFARS)

Time 5 minutes

Ages 7–18

Time Frame Not specified

Purpose Assessment of positive and negative affect and physiological arousal.

Commentary

The AFARS was designed to assess factors of the tripartite model of emotion.

Versions

The Affect and Arousal Scale (AFARS) is only available as a self-report form.

Properties

Items   The AFARS comprises 27 items that are rated on a 4-point scale with responses: never true, sometimes true, most times true, and always true.

Scales   Factor analysis was used to investigate the structure of the AFARS, which revealed three factors. The items are scored on the three scales which are labeled Positive Affect, Negative Affect, and Physical Arousal.

Reliability   Test–retest correlations across a 1-week interval were 0.68 for Positive Affect, 0.68 for Negative Affect, and 0.72 for Physical Arousal.

Cronbach's alphas were 0.80 for Positive Affect, 0.77 for Negative Affect, and 0.81 for Physical Arousal.

Validity   The Positive Affect scale correlated negatively with depressive symptom and did not correlate with anxiety symptoms. The Negative Affect scale correlated positively with depressive and anxiety symptoms. The physical Arousal scale correlated positively with other physiological measures and correlated moderately with depressive and anxiety symptoms.

Norms   Means and standard deviations of the AFARS scales are available for 1589 children in grades 3 through 12 from Hawaii.

Use   No supplementary materials available.

Key references

Chorpita BF, Daleiden EL, Moffitt C, Yim L, Umemoto LA. Assessment of tripartite factors of emotion in children and adolescents I: Structural validity and normative data of an Affect and Arousal Scale. J Psychopathol Behav Assess 2000; 22: 141–60.

Daleiden EL, Chorpita BF, Lu W. Assessment of tripartite factors of emotion in children and adolescents II: Concurrent validity of the Affect and Arousal Scale for children. J Psychopathol Behav Assess 2000; 22: 161–82.

Address

Bruce F. Chorpita
Department of Psychology
University of Hawaii at Manoa
2430 Campus Road
Honolulu, HI 96822
USA
chorpita@hawaii.edu

The Affect and Arousal Scale (AFARS)

Directions. This form is about how you feel. For each sentence that you read, circle the answer that best tells how true that sentence is about how you usually feel. Remember, there are no right or wrong answers, just circle what you think describes you best.

1. When I'm doing well at something, I really feel good.	never true	sometimes true	most times true	always true
2. Other people upset me.	never true	sometimes true	most times true	always true
3. Often I have trouble getting my breath.	never true	sometimes true	most times true	always true
4. I get upset easily.	never true	sometimes true	most times true	always true
5. My mouth gets dry.	never true	sometimes true	most times true	always true
6. I have fun at school.	never true	sometimes true	most times true	always true
7. My heart beats too fast.	never true	sometimes true	most times true	always true
8. Little things bother me.	never true	sometimes true	most times true	always true
9. I will try something new if I think it will be fun.	never true	sometimes true	most times true	always true
10. My hands get shaky.	never true	sometimes true	most times true	always true
11. When I get something I want, I feel excited.	never true	sometimes true	most times true	always true
12. I over-react to things.	never true	sometimes true	most times true	always true
13. I have trouble swallowing.	never true	sometimes true	most times true	always true
14. I love going to new places.	never true	sometimes true	most times true	always true
15. I get upset by little things.	never true	sometimes true	most times true	always true
16. I feel shaky.	never true	sometimes true	most times true	always true
17. I would love to win a contest.	never true	sometimes true	most times true	always true
18. I don't like to wait for things.	never true	sometimes true	most times true	always true
19. I like being with people.	never true	sometimes true	most times true	always true
20. I have trouble breathing.	never true	sometimes true	most times true	always true
21. When I see a chance for fun, I take it.	never true	sometimes true	most times true	always true
22. I get upset.	never true	sometimes true	most times true	always true
23. When good things happen to me, I feel full of energy.	never true	sometimes true	most times true	always true
24. I have plenty of friends.	never true	sometimes true	most times true	always true
25. I sometimes feel faint.	never true	sometimes true	most times true	always true
26. I can't calm down once I am upset.	never true	sometimes true	most times true	always true
27. Often I feel sick in my stomach.	never true	sometimes true	most times true	always true

Childhood Anxiety Sensitivity Index (CASI)

Time 5 minutes

Ages 8–15

Time Frame Not specified

Purpose Assessment of belief that anxiety symptoms have negative consequences.

Commentary

The CASI is an adaptation of the Anxiety Sensitivity Index (ASI) for adults (Reiss et al., 1986).

Versions

The childhood Anxiety Sensitivity Index (CASI) is available only as a self-report form.

Properties

Items The CASI comprises 18 items that are rated on a 3-point scale with responses: none, some, and a lot.

Scales The items of the CASI are scored on the total anxiety sensitivity score which is the sum of all items.

Reliability Test–retest correlations for the total anxiety sensitivity score were 0.76 across a 2-week interval among school children and 0.79 across a 1-week interval among clinical children.

Cronbach's alphas for the total anxiety sensitivity score were both 0.87 on two occasions among school children and 0.87 among clinical children.

Validity Correlations of the total anxiety sensitivity score of the CASI among school children were 0.74 and 0.64 with a self-report measure of phobic fears, 0.30 and 0.51 with a self-report measure of anxiety frequency on two occasions, and 0.64 with a self-report measure of trait anxiety. Correlations among clinical children were 0.59 with self-reported phobic fears, 0.12 with self-reported anxiety frequency, and 0.62 with self-reported trait anxiety.

Norms Tables with means and standard deviations of the CASI total anxiety sensitivity scores of 85 school children and 33 clinical children are given in Silverman et al. (1991).

Use No supplementary materials available.

Key references

Reiss S, Peterson RA, Gursky DM, McNally RJ. Anxiety sensitivity, anxiety frequency and the prediction of fearfulness. Behav Res Ther 1986; 24: 1–8.

Silverman WK, Fleisig W, Rabian B, Peterson RA. Childhood Anxiety Sensitivity Index. J Clin Child Psychol 1991; 20: 162–8.

Address

Wendy K. Silverman
Child and Family Psychosocial Research Center
Child Anxiety and Phobia Program
Department of Psychology
University Park
Florida International University
Miami, FL 33199
USA
silverw@fiu.edu

Childhood Anxiety Sensitivity Index (CASI)

Directions: A number of statements which boys and girls use to describe themselves are given below. Read each statement carefully and put an X on the line in front of the words that describe you. There are no right or wrong answers. Remember, find the words that best describe you.

Name: _____ Age: _____ Date: _____

1.	I don't want other people to know when I feel afraid	___ None	___ Some	___ A lot
2.	When I cannot keep my mind on my schoolwork, I worry that I might be going crazy	___ None	___ Some	___ A lot
3.	It scares me when I feel 'shaky'	___ None	___ Some	___ A lot
4.	It scares me when I feel like I am going to faint	___ None	___ Some	___ A lot
5.	It is important for me to stay in control of my feelings	___ None	___ Some	___ A lot
6.	It scares me when my heart beats fast	___ None	___ Some	___ A lot
7.	It embarrasses me when my stomach growls (makes noises)	___ None	___ Some	___ A lot
8.	It scares me when I feel like I am going to throw up	___ None	___ Some	___ A lot
9.	When I notice that my heart is beating fast, I worry that there might be something wrong with me	___ None	___ Some	___ A lot
10.	It scares me when I have trouble getting my breath	___ None	___ Some	___ A lot
11.	When my stomach hurts, I worry that I might be really sick	___ None	___ Some	___ A lot
12.	It scares me when I can't keep my mind on my schoolwork	___ None	___ Some	___ A lot
13.	Other kids can tell when I feel shaky	___ None	___ Some	___ A lot
14.	Unusual feelings in my body scare me	___ None	___ Some	___ A lot
15.	When I am afraid, I worry that I might be crazy	___ None	___ Some	___ A lot
16.	It scares me when I feel nervous	___ None	___ Some	___ A lot
17.	I don't like to let my feelings show	___ None	___ Some	___ A lot
18.	Funny feelings in my body scare me	___ None	___ Some	___ A lot

Fear Survey Schedule for Children – Revised (FSSC-R)

Time 15 minutes

Ages 7–16

Time Frame Not specified

Purpose Assessment of phobic fears.

Commentary

The FSSC-R is an adaptation of Scherer and Nakamura's Fear Survey Schedule for Children (1968) and was designed as an instrument for identifying specific fears in children and adolescents, selecting fearful children and adolescents for prevention and treatment trials, and determining pre-treatment and post-treatment differences in therapy outcome studies. The FSSC-R has been used in applied and research settings and is especially useful as an instrument for assessing specific feared situations or objects that lead to avoidance behaviors in children and adolescents with specific phobias and social phobias.

Versions

The Fear Survey Schedule for Children-Revised (FSSC-R) was designed as a self-report form, but a later developed parent-report form is available as well.

Properties

Items   The FSSC-R comprises 80 items that are rated on a 3-point scale with responses: none, some, and a lot.

Scales   Factor analysis supported five factors. Therefore, the items are scored on five subscales which are labeled: Failure and Criticism, The Unknown, Minor Injury and Small Animals, Danger and Death, and Medical Fears, and on the total score, which is the simple sum of all items. In addition, the number of items that are endorsed with response 'a lot' is denoted the frequency score.

Reliability   Test–retest correlations were 0.82 across a 1-week interval, 0.87 across a 2-week interval, and 0.62 across a 3-month interval for the total score. Test–retest correlations across a 3-month interval ranged from 0.70 to 0.87 for the 5 subscales.

Cronbach's alphas were consistently above 0.90 for the total score and ranged from 0.57 to 0.89 for the subscales in several samples.

Validity   The total score and subscales of the FSSC-R correlated significantly with several measures of self-reported anxiety. However, the correlations among anxiety measures were higher than correlations with the FSSC-R, which indicated that the FSSC-R assessed other aspects of anxiety, i.e. phobic fears, than the other measures of anxiety.

Discriminant analysis revealed that the FSSC-R total and subscale scores differentiated well among clinical children diagnosed with simple phobias of animals, dark or sleeping alone, shots or doctors, and social phobia.

Norms   Tables with means and standard deviations separated by sex and age groups of the total score and subscale scores of normal children from the USA and Australia are given in Ollendick, King and Frary (1989).

Use   A short manual, scoring instructions that include normative data, and a copy of the scale can be obtained from Thomas H. Ollendick at the address below. The FSSC-R has been translated into several languages.

Key references

Ollendick TH, King NJ, Frary RB. Fears in children and adolescents: Reliability and generalizability across gender, age and nationality. Behav Res Ther 1989; 27: 19–26.

Muris P, Merckelbach P, Ollendick T, King N, Bogie N. Three traditional and three new childhood anxiety questionnaires: Their reliability and validity in a normal adolescent sample. Behav Res Ther 2002; 40: 753–72.

Ollendick TH. Reliability and validity of the Revised Fear Survey Schedule for Children (FSSC-R). Behav Res Ther 1983; 21: 685–92.

Scherer MW, Nakamura CY. A Fear Survey Schedule for Children (FSS-FC): A factor analytic comparison with manifest anxiety (CMAS). Behav Res Ther 1968; 6: 173–82.

Kutcher Generalized Social Anxiety Disorder Scale for Adolescents (K-GSADS-A)

Time 15 minutes

Ages 11–17

Time Frame Not specified

Purpose Assessment of social anxiety problems.

Commentary

The K-GSADS-A was specifically designed to assess treatment outcome for adolescents. It is especially useful for monitoring severity of symptoms over time. At the time of its development no clinician-rated scales were available for assessing severity of social phobia in children or adolescents.

Versions

The Kutcher Generalized Social Anxiety Disorder Scale for Adolescents (K-GSADS-A) is only available as a clinician-rated scale.

Properties

Items The K-GSADS-A comprises 3 sections. The first section comprises 18 items pertaining to fear and avoidance of social situations. The items are rated on two 4-point scales for indicating discomfort/anxiety/distress with responses from none to severe, and for indicating avoidance with responses from none to total avoidance. The second section asks for the respondent's three most feared social situations which are then rated on the same 4-point scales as items from the first section. The third section comprises 11 items pertaining to affective and somatic distress. These items are scored on a 4-point scale with responses: never, mild, moderate, and severe.

Scales The items of the first and third sections yield 4 subscale scores which are labeled: Fear and Anxiety, Avoidance, Affective Distress, and Somatic Distress. In addition, the Total Score is the sum of the 4 subscales.

Reliability Test–retest intraclass correlation across a 4-week interval was 0.64 among adolescents in the placebo condition of a 16-week trial.

Cronbach's alphas averaged across 5 assessments in a 16-week trial were 0.92 for Fear and Anxiety, 0.91 for Avoidance, 0.86 for Affective Distress, 0.74 for Somatic Distress, and 0.96 for the Total Score.

Validity Correlations at 5 time points of a 16-week trial of the K-GSADS-A Total Score with another clinician-rated measure of social anxiety and self-rated social anxiety ranged from 0.56 to 0.94. Absolute values of correlations with clinician-rated functioning ranged from 0.26 to 0.69. Correlations with clinician-rated depression were lower than with anxiety. All correlations were significant and increased across the 5 time points.

Baseline Total Score and subscale scores were not significantly different between adolescents in the treatment and placebo conditions in a 16-week psychopharmacotherapy trial, while postbaseline scores significantly distinguished the treatment and placebo groups.

Norms No information available.

Use Copies of the K-GSADS-A can be obtained from Stan Kutcher at the address listed below.

Key references

Brooks SJ, Kutcher S. The Kutcher Generalized Social Anxiety Disorder Scale for Adolescents: Assessment of its evaluative properties over the course of a 16-week pediatric psychopharmacotherapy trial. J Child Adolesc Psychopharmacol 2004; 14: 273–86.

Address

Stan Kutcher
Department of Psychiatry
Dalhousie University, QE II HSC
Abbie J. Lane Building
Suite 9212
5909 Veteran's Memorial Lane
Halifax, Nova Scotia B3H 2E2
Canada
stan.kutcher@dal.ca

Kutcher Generalised Social Anxiety Disorder Scale for Adolescents (K-GSADS-A)

Section A: Fear and avoidance   (0 = none; 3 = severe/total avoidance)

Item		Discomfort, anxiety, distress (0–3)	Avoidance (0–3)
1	Initiating conversation with a member of the opposite sex		
2	Attending a party or other social gathering with people you don't know very well		
3	Speaking up, answering questions in class/participating in class discussions		
4	Presenting in front of a small group or in a classroom setting		
5	Attending overnight group activities such as camps, school trips, etc.		
6	Speaking to a store clerk, bank teller, etc.		
7	Asking a stranger for directions		
8	Changing in a common locker room		
9	Showering in a common shower room		
10	Using a public toilet facility or urinating in public (score whatever is greater)		
11	Telephoning to ask for information or to speak to someone you don't know very well (score whatever is greater)		
12	Entering a classroom or social group once the class or activity is already underway		
13	Initiating conversation with strangers		
14	Speaking with authority figures: i.e. teachers, counselor, principal, police officers, clergy, physician, etc.		
15	Eating in public		
16	Going to a party alone		
17	Asking someone for a date		
18	Writing your name in public		

Section B Fear/avoidance: seminal items

What are your three most feared social situations and how strong is the fear/avoidance of each (0 = none; 3 = severe/total avoidance)?

		Fear	Avoidance
1	_____		
2	_____		
3	_____		

Section C: Distress quotient

In general, how strongly do these items occur to you in most social situations?

Scoring: 0 = Never   1 = Mild   2 = Moderate   3 = Severe

Item		Score (0–3)
1	Feeling embarrassed or humiliated	
2	Feeling 'centered out', scrutinized by others	
3	Feeling judged or critically evaluated by others	
4	Wanting to leave the social situation	
5	Anxious anticipation of social situation	
6	Experiences a panic attack	
7	Blushes	
8	Sweats or hot/cold flashes	
9	Urination urges	
10	Gastrointestinal distress	
11	Trembling or shaking	

Subscale scores and total score:

SS1: Fear and Anxiety Score (Items A 1–18, anxiety column)
SS2: Avoidance Score (Items A 1–18, avoidance column)
SS3: Affective Distress Score (Items C 1–5)
SS4: Somatic Distress Score (Items C 6–11)

Total K-GSADS-A Score (SS1 + SS2 + SS3 + SS4)

Interpretation of scores:
There are no validated diagnostic categories associated with particular ranges of scores. All scores should be assessed relative to an individual patient's baseline score (higher scores indicating worsening social phobia, lower scores suggesting possible improvement).

Liebowitz Social Anxiety Scale for Children and Adolescents (LSAS-CA)

Time 10 minutes

Ages 7–18

Time Frame Not specified

Purpose Assessment of social anxiety and avoidance.

Commentary

The LSAS-CA is based on the Liebowitz Social Anxiety Scale for Adults.

Versions

The Liebowitz Social Anxiety Scale for Children and Adolescents (LSAS-CA) is only available as a clinician's rating scale.

Properties

Items   The LSAS-CA comprises 24 items describing 12 social interaction and 12 performance situations. The items are rated on two 4-point scales: 1) an anxiety scale with responses: none, mild, moderate; 2) an avoidance scale with responses: never (0%), sometimes (1–33%), often (34–67%), and usually (68–100%).

Scales   The items of the LSAS-CA are scored on two anxiety scales labeled: Interaction anxiety and Performance interaction, and on two avoidance scales: Interaction avoidance and Performance avoidance. In addition, Total anxiety is the sum of the two anxiety scales, Total avoidance is the sum of the two avoidance scales, and Total Score is the sum of Total anxiety and Total avoidance.

Reliability   Test–retest intraclass correlations across a 3- to 7-day interval ranged from 0.89 to 0.94.

   Cronbach's alphas ranged from 0.90 to 0.97.

Validity   The LSAS-CA was correlated with measures of social anxiety, depression, impairment, and functioning. Correlations were highest between LSAS-CA and social phobia measures. Correlations were moderate between LSAS-CA and impairment and functioning measures, and lowest between LSAS-CA and depression measures.

   Analyses of variance revealed significant differences of LSAS-CA scores among three groups of children: children with social phobia had the highest scores, children with mixed anxiety diagnoses had the next highest scores, and nonpsychiatric children had the lowest scores.

   A cut-off point of 22.5 for the total score distinguished between children with social phobia and nonpsychiatric children with a sensitivity of 96% and a specificity of 100%.

Norms   A cut-off point has been reported in Masia-Warner et al (2003).

Use   A manual and copies of the LSAS-CA are available from Carrie Masia-Warner at the address below.

Key references

Masia-Warner C, Storch EA, Pincus DB, et al. The Liebowitz Social Anxiety Scale for Children and Adolescents: An initial psychometric investigation. J Am Acad Child Adolesc Psychiatry 2003; 42: 1076–84.

Address

Carrie Masia-Warner
NYU Child Study Center
215 Lexington Avenue, 13th Floor
New York, NY 10016
USA
carrie.masia@med.nyu.edu

Multidimensional Anxiety Scale for Children (MASC)

Time 15 minutes

Ages 8–19

Time Frame Not specified

Purpose Assessment of anxiety problems.

Commentary

The MASC was developed to assess the major dimensions of anxiety that are specific for children and adolescents. Anxiety rating scales that were available were often downward extensions of adult scales, did not match DSM-IV criteria, and did not assess multiple dimensions of anxiety. The MASC was developed to address these shortcomings.

Versions

The Multidimensional Anxiety Scale for Children (MASC) is only available as self-report. The MASC comes in two lengths: the standard version comprises 39 items and the short version 10 items.

Properties

Items The MASC comprises 39 items that are rated on a 4-point scale with responses: never true about me, rarely true about me, sometimes true about me, and often true about me.

Scales Factor analysis was used to determine the scale structure of the MASC. Four basic scales were derived. Next, for each scale, the items constituting these scales were subjected to factor analysis. The analyses revealed that three of the basic scales could be further divided into two subscales. The basic scales and their accompanying subscales are: Physical Symptoms with subscales Tense/Restless and Somatic/Autonomic, Harm Avoidance with subscales Perfectionism and Anxious Coping, Social Anxiety with Humiliation/Rejection and Performance Fears, and Separation/Panic. In addition, the simple sum of all item ratings constitutes the Total Anxiety scale. Furthermore, two additional indices are available: the Anxiety Disorders Index for distinguishing between children and adolescents with and without anxiety disorders, and the Inconsistency Index for detecting response bias.

Reliability Test–retest correlations for the basic scales and subscales across a 3-month interval ranged from 0.70 to 0.93 among children and adolescents with an anxiety disorder or an attention-deficit/hyperactivity disorder.

Cronbach's alphas for the basic scales and subscales across sex and age groups ranged from 0.46 to 0.89 among children and adolescents recruited from elementary, junior high and high schools.

Validity The basic scales Physical Symptoms, Harm Avoidance, Social Anxiety, Separation/Panic, and Total Anxiety correlated 0.71, –0.13, 0.55, 0.43, and 0.63, respectively with self-reported anxiety and 0.34, –0.32, 0.14, 0.25, and 0.19, respectively among clinical children and adolescents.

Discriminant analysis was used to test whether the four basic scales Physical Symptoms, Harm Avoidance, Social Anxiety, Separation/Panic, and Total Anxiety were able to distinguish between children and adolescents diagnosed with anxiety disorder and those without disorders. The analysis revealed that the four scales could discriminate between the two groups with a sensitivity of 90% and a specificity of 84%. The Anxiety Disorders Index discriminated between children and adolescents with an anxiety disorder and those without disorders with a sensitivity of 83% and a specificity of 92%, and between children and adolescents with an anxiety disorder and those with an attention-deficit/hyperactivity disorder with a sensitivity of 75% and a specificity of 67%.

Norms The MASC was standardized on the ratings of 2698 children and adolescents aged 8–19 years recruited from elementary, junior high and high schools. Norms are separated by sex and three age groups: 8–11 years, 12–15 years, and 16–19 years. Raw scores are converted to T-scores.

Use A manual and rating scales enabling direct scoring, a manual, a computer program for data entry and scoring are available from the publisher at the address below.

Key references

March JS. MASC Multidimensional Anxiety Scale for Children. North Tonawanda, NY: Multi-Health Systems Inc, 1997.

March JS, Parker JDA, Sullivan K, Stallings P, Conners CK. The Multidimensional Anxiety Scale for Children MASC): Factor structure, reliability and validity. J Am Acad Child Adolesc Psychiatry 1997; 36: 554–65.

March JS, Sullivan K, Parker JDA. Test–retest reliability of the Multidimensional Anxiety Scale for Children. J Anxiety Dis 1999; 13: 349–58.

Address

Multi-Health Systems Inc.
P.O. Box 950
North Tonawanda, NY 14120–0950
USA
www.mhs.com

Multidimensional Anxiety Scale for Children (MASC) – sample items

	Never true about me	Rarely true about me	Sometimes true about me	Often true about me
4. I get scared when my parents go away	0	1	2	3
14. I worry about getting called on in class	0	1	2	3
19. I avoid going to places without my family	0	1	2	3
22. I worry about what other people think of me	0	1	2	3
27. I feel restless and on edge	0	1	2	3
33. I get nervous if I have to perform in public	0	1	2	3

Pediatric Anxiety Rating Scale (PARS)

Time 30 minutes

Ages 6–17

Time Frame Last week

Purpose Assessment of the severity of anxiety symptoms.

Commentary

No clinician-rated instruments existed for assessing both impairment and overall anxiety impaired in youths prior to the PARS. The PARS was developed to fill this gap and was modeled after similar instruments for assessing the severity and impairment of obsessive-compulsive symptoms and tics.

Versions

The Pediatric Anxiety Rating Scale (PARS) is a clinician's rating scale.

Properties

Items   The PARS has two sections: a symptom checklist and severity items. The symptom checklist comprises 50 items to determine anxiety symptoms during the previous week. The items are rated on a 2-point scale with responses: yes and no. In addition, the PARS comprises seven items to determine the severity of the anxiety symptoms. The items are rated on a 6-point scale with different anchors for each item.

Scales   The severity items form seven dimensions: (1) number of symptoms, (2) frequency of symptoms, (3) severity of distress associated with anxiety symptoms, (4) severity of physical symptoms, (5) avoidance, (6) interference at home, (7) interference out of home. The sum of five severity items constitutes the PARS Total Score. Number of symptoms and physical symptoms were not included in the sum.

Reliability   Test–retest intra-class correlations across a 1- to 4-week interval ranged from 0.35 to 0.59 for the severity items and was 0.55 for the PARS Total Score.

Interrater intra-class correlations across raters ranged from 0.78 to 0.96 for the severity items and was 0.97 for the PARS Total Score.

Cronbach's alpha for the five items comprising the PARS Total Score was 0.64.

Validity   The PARS Total Score correlated moderately with clinician- and parent-reported measures of anxiety and lower, but still significant, with self-reported anxiety. Correlations of the PARS Total Score with measures of depression were small, but significant.

The PARS showed a reduction in severity from pre- to post-treatment. The change in PARS scores correlated with changes in other global severity ratings and specific anxiety symptoms of some but not all measures.

Norms   No information available.

Use   No supplemental materials available.

Key references

The research units on pediatric psychopharmacology anxiety study group. The Pediatric Anxiety Rating Scale (PARS): Development and psychometric properties. J Am Acad Child Adolesc Psychiatry 2002; 41: 1061–9

Address

Mark A. Riddle
Division of Child and Adolescent Psychiatry
Johns Hopkins Children's Center
Room 346
600 North Wolfe Street
Baltimore, MD 21287–3325
USA
mriddle@jhmi.edu

Version 1.2 July 11, 1997

This instrument was developed by the Research Units of Pediatric Psychopharmacology (RUPPs) at Johns Hopkins Medical Institutions, Mark A. Riddle, M.D., PI, and at the College of Physicians and Surgeons, Columbia University, Laurence L. Greenhill, PI. This effort was funded by the National Institute of Mental Health, Benedetto Vitiello, M.D., Project Officer. Helpful consultation was provided by Prudence Fisher, Ph.D., Columbia University.

Please obtain permission to use, copy or cite this instrument from Dr. Riddle (410.955.2320) or Dr. Greenhill (212.960.2340).

Instructions

Overview: The Pediatric Anxiety Rating Scale (PARS) is to be used to rate the severity of anxiety in children and adolescents, ages 6 to 17 years. The PARS has two sections: the symptom checklist and the severity items. The symptom checklist is used to determine the child's repertoire of symptoms during the past week. The 7-severity item is used to determine severity of symptoms and the PARS total score.

Symptoms include in the rating are commonly observed in patients with the following disorder, panic disorder and specific phobia. Obviously, there is considerable overlap in symptoms among these anxiety disorders. Symptoms specific to obsessive compulsive disorder and post traumatic stress disorder are not included.

The time frame for the PARS rating is the past week. Only those symptoms endorsed for the past week are included in the symptom checklist and rated on the severity items.

The respondents should be the same for each rating on the same subject. For example, in a treatment trial, where the PARS may be administered multiple times to the same child, it is important that the same primary caregiver (e.g., mother) be present at each rating. If both parents are present for the first rating, both should be present for subsequent ratings.

The format of the interview: The goal of the interview is to elicit as much information as possible about the child's level of anxiety. To achieve this goal, it is necessary to obtain information from both the child and the primary caregiver (at least). The clinician combines all information from all informants to make the ratings.

Usually, for pre-teens, the interviewer starts with the parent(s) alone and subsequently interviews the child alone. For teenagers, the reverse order is generally preferred (adolescent first, followed by the parent(s)). With some families, it may be preferable to interview the child and parent(s) together. Both should be told in advance that they will have an opportunity, if indicated, to speak alone with the interviewer. The order and procedure for interviews should remain constant throughout multiple ratings.

Symptom Checklist: The symptom checklist is the first of the two major sections of the PARS. The goal of the checklist is to document the array of the patient's symptoms that will be used to establish severity during the ratings of severity items. Thus, the symptom checklist is not to be used to establish severity.

Use items as probes to elicit the patient's complete symptom repertoire. Elicit information from both child and parent(s). Use your best judgement to combine information from all informants. Remember, symptoms occurring during the past week only are to be recorded.

Severity Ratings: Using all of the symptoms endorsed for the past week, rate severity of symptoms for each of the 7 severity items. Use the anchors for each item to assist the child and parent in establishing severity. Respondents may wonder whether the severity items are rating an average for the past week, or the worst day, or worst time, etc. The severity items are meant to elicit information about average symptom severity over the past week. Record all scores in whole numbers; in-between scores (e.g., 1.5) are not permitted.

Follow-up Evaluations: Eliciting information about the symptom list can be much more efficient during subsequent ratings of the same subject. The interviewer can use the symptom checklist from the prior rating as a guide. For a follow-up rating, the interviewer can describe to the subject the symptoms that were endorsed at the prior rating. Then the interviewer asks if there have been any new symptoms during the past week. Finally, the interviewer uses the probes to be sure that no symptoms have been overlooked. However, since the subject will be familiar with the probes from prior assessments, the probes can be reviewed rapidly, with the expectation that they will not be endorsed.

Scoring: The total score for the PARS is total of the 7 severity items. The total score ranges from 0 to 35. (Codes '8' and '9' are not included in the summation.) For clinical trials, severity is based on the sum of items #2,3,5,6, and 7.

Sample Probes for the Symptom List: Social interactions or performance situations: During the past week, have you (has s/he) worried about or avoided social situaitons? Let me give you some examples (refer to list). During the past week, have you (has s/he) been shy about or refused to do things in public? Let me give you some more examples.

Separation Anxiety: Some children worry about being away from their mother or father. What about you (your child)? Some children do things to make sure they stay near their mother or father? What about you (your child)? Let me give you examples.

Generalized Anxiety: Some people worry about a lot of different things. What about you (your child)? What about during the past week? Let me give you some examples.

Specific Phobia: Do you worry about or have fears of animals (e.g. dog), etc?

Physical Signs/Symptoms: Sometimes children notice feelings or changes in their bodies when they are anxious or worried? What about you? Let me give examples.

Symptom checklist

Instructions: Fill in the blanks with '1' (yes), '2' (no), or '9' (other, e.g., unable or unwilling to answer)

Social interactions or performance situations	Parent	Child	Rater
1. Has fear of and/or avoids participating in group activities	____	____	____
2. Has fear of and/or avoids going to a party or social event	____	____	____
3. Has fear of and/or avoids talking with a stranger	____	____	____
4. Has fear of and/or avoids talking on the phone	____	____	____
5. Reluctant or refuses to talk in front of a group	____	____	____
6. Reluctant or refuses to write in front of other people	____	____	____
7. Reluctant or refuses to eat in public.	____	____	____
8. Reluctant or refuses to use a public bathroom.	____	____	____
9. Reluctant or refuses to change into gym clothes or bathing suit with others present.	____	____	____

Separation			
10. Worry about harm happening to attachment figures	____	____	____
11. Worry about harm befalling self, including the fear of dying	____	____	____
12. Distress when separation occurs or is anticipated	____	____	____
13. Fear or reluctance to be alone	____	____	____
14. Reluctance or refusal to go to school or elsewhere	____	____	____
15. Complaints of physical symptoms when separation occurs or is anticipated	____	____	____
16. Reluctance or refusal to go to sleep alone	____	____	____
17. Reluctance or refusal to sleep away from home	____	____	____
18. Nightmares with a separation theme	____	____	____
19. Clings to parent, or follows parent around the house	____	____	____

Generalized			
20. Excessive worry about everyday or real-life problems	____	____	____
21. Restlessness or feeling keyed-up or on edge	____	____	____
22. Easily fatigued	____	____	____
23. Difficulty concentrating or mind going blank	____	____	____
24. Irritability	____	____	____
25. Muscle tension or nonspecific tension	____	____	____
26. Sleep disturbance, especially difficulty falling asleep	____	____	____
27. Dread or fearful anticipation (nonspecific)	____	____	____

Specific phobia			
28. Animal: Specify			
29. Natural environment: (e.g., heights, storms) Specify:	____	____	____
30. Blood-injection-injury: Specify:	____	____	____
31. Situational (e.g., airplane, elevator): Specify:	____	____	____

Acute physical signs and symptoms			
32. Blushing	____	____	____
33. Feels paralyzed	____	____	____
34. Trembling or shaking	____	____	____
35. Feels dizzy, unsteady, lightheaded or going to pass out	____	____	____
36. Palpitations or pounding heart	____	____	____
37. Difficult breathing (sensation of shortness of breath, smothering or choking)	____	____	____
38. Chills or hot flashes	____	____	____
39. Sweating	____	____	____
40. Feels sick to stomach, nausea or abdominal distress	____	____	____
41. Recurrent urge to go to bathroom	____	____	____
42. Chest pain or discomfort	____	____	____
43. Paresthesias (numbness or tingling sensation in fingers, toes, or perioral region)	____	____	____
44. Problems swallowing or eating	____	____	____

Other			
45. Crying spells when in anxiety-provoking situations	____	____	____
46. Temper tantrums when in anxiety-provoking situations	____	____	____
47. Needs to flee certain anxiety-provoking situations	____	____	____
48. Keeps distance from other people	____	____	____
49. Fear of losing control or going crazy	____	____	____
50. Derealization (feeling of unreality) or depersonalization (detached from oneself)	____	____	____

Other anxiety symptoms: Specify: _____

Specify: _____

Specify: _____

Severity items

Instructions: For each item circle the number that best characterizes the patient during the past week.

1. Overall number of anxiety symptoms (circle code for past week only)   Code

Not applicable	8
Does not know	9
No symptoms	0
1 symptom	1
2-3 symptoms	2
4-6 symptoms	3
7-10 symptoms	4
More than 10 symptoms	5

2. Overall frequency of anxiety symptoms

Not applicable	8
Does not know	9
No symptoms	0
1 or 2 days a week	1
3 or 4 days a week	2
5 or 6 days a week	3
Daily	4
Several hours every day	5

3. Overall severity of anxiety feelings

	Not applicable	8
	Does not know.	9
	None. No anxious symptoms.	0
Minimal:	Very transient discomfort. Not clinically significant.	1
Mild:	Transient discomfort that is mildly disturbing. Borderline clinical significance. Intermediate between 1and 3.	2
Moderate:	Clearly nervous when anticipating or confronting the anxiety-provoking situation(s). Often unable to overcome these feelings. These feelings impact on well-being.	3
Severe:	Very distressed when anxious or when anticipating or confronting the anxiety-provoking situation (s). Usually unable to overcome this feeling. Intermediate between 3 and 5.	4
Extreme:	Feels wretched when anticipating or confronting anxiety-provoking situation(s). Often or almost totally unable to overcome this fear. Very marked impact on well being.	5

4. Overall severity of physical symptoms of anxiety

	Not applicable	8
	Does not know	9
	None. No physical symptoms of anxiety.	0
Minimal:	Very transient physical symptoms of anxiety. Symptoms are not, or are hardly noticeable by others. Not clinically significant.	1
Mild:	Few physical symptoms: no lasting impact. Borderline clinical significance. Intermediate between 1and 3.	2
Moderate:	Persistent physical symptoms of anxiety, especially during exposure to the feared situation(s). Symptoms are noticeable by others and significantly interfere with his/her ability to function in the situation.	3
Severe:	Marked physical symptoms of substantial clinical significance. Intermediate between 3 and 5.	4
Extreme:	Severe and persistent physical symptoms of anxiety, especially during exposure to the feared situations(s). Symptoms are very obvious to others and often result in inability to function in the situation.	5

5. Overall avoidance of anxiety-provoking situations

NOTE: Rate all avoidance here; include school, home, activities, etc. in rating

	Not applicable	8
	Does not know	9
	None. Does not avoid the anxiety-provoking situation(s).	0
Minimal:	Very occasionally avoids the anxiety-provoking situation(s). Avoided situation(s) is/are not critical to his/her well-being.	1
Mild:	Avoids anxiety-provoking situation(s) some of the time but no important situation is consistently avoided. Borderline clinical significance. Intermediate between 1 and 3.	2
Moderate:	Avoid anxiety-provoking situation(s) frequently. At least one important situation is avoided.	3
Severe:	Avoids anxiety-provoking situation most of the time or more than one important situation is consistently avoided. Intermediate between 3 and 5.	4
Extreme:	Avoids all or almost all anxiety-provoking situations.	5

6. Interference with family relationships and/or performance at home

	Not applicable	8
	Does not know	9
	None. No interference.	0
Minimal:	Very transient interference. No impact on relationships with family members or performance (tasks, etc.) at home.	1
Mild:	Slight impact on relationships or performance outside of the home. Borderline clinical significance. Intermediate between 1 and 3.	2
Moderate:	Clear interference. Either performance of tasks at home or frequency or quality of interaction with family members is affected: he/she might withdraw from interaction, or might be avoided/rejected by family members, or might have many conflicts with them.	3
Severe:	Marked interference in relationships with family members and/or performance at home. Of substantial clinical significance. Intermediate between 3 and 5.	4
Extreme:	Totally or almost totally unable to maintain appropriate family relationship and/or function at home.	5

7. Interference with peer and adult relationships and/or performance outside of home.

NOTE: Out-of-home functioning includes school (not avoidance), activities, etc

	Not applicable	8
	Does not know	9
	None. No interference.	0
Minimal:	Very transient interference. No impact on relationships with peers or teachers or other adults outside of the home. No impact on functioning outside of home, e.g., attending and performing group activities.	1
Mild:	Slight impact on relationships or performance outside of the home. Borderline clinical significance. Intermediate between 1 and 3.	2
Moderate:	Clear interference. Either performance outside of the home or frequency or quality of peer or adult interactions is affected: he/she might withdraw from interaction, or might be avoided/rejected by peers or adults, or might have conflicts with them.	3
Severe:	Marked interference in relationship with peers or adults outside of home and/or performance outside of home. Of substantial clinical significance. Intermediate between 3 and 5.	4
Extreme:	Totally or almost totally unable to maintain appropriate peer or adult relationship and/or function outside of home.	5

Penn State Worry Questionnaire for Children (PSWQ-C)

Time 5 minutes

Ages 6–18

Time Frame Not specified

Purpose Assessment of worry.

Commentary

The PSWQ-C is an adaptation of the Penn State Worry Questionnaire for adults (Meyer et al., 1990).

Versions

The Penn State Worry Questionnaire for Children (PSWQ-C) is only available as a self-report form.

Properties

Items   The PSWQ-C comprises 14 items that are rated on a 4-point scale with responses: never true, sometimes true, most times true, always true.

Scales   Factor analysis of the items of the PSWQ-C revealed that a one-factor solution was adequate, so that the items are scored on a total score scale.

Reliability   Test–retest correlation across a 1-week interval was 0.92.

Cronbach's alphas were 0.81 for 6–11-year-olds and 0.90 for 12–18-year-olds.

Validity   The PSWQ-C correlated high with another self-report measure of worry and this correlation was significantly higher than correlations of the PSWQ-C with self-report measures of anxiety and depression.

Children diagnosed with generalized anxiety disorder had significantly higher scores than children diagnosed with other anxiety disorders. Both groups of children with anxiety disorders had significantly higher scores than non-referred children with no mental disorder.

Norms   A table with means and standard deviations of PSWQ-C scores of 199 6–18-year-old children can be found in Chorpita et al. (1997).

Use   No supplemental materials available.

Key references

Chorpita BF, Tracey SA, Brown TA, Collica TJ, Barlow DH. Assessment of worry in children an adolescents: An adaptation of the Penn State Worry Questionnaire. Behav Res Ther 1997; 35: 569–81.

Meyer TJ, Miller ML, Metzger RL, Borkovec TD. Development and validation of the Penn State Worry Questionnaire. Behav Res Ther 1990; 28: 487–95.

Muris P, Meesters C, Gobel M. Reliability, validity, and normative data of the Penn State Worry Questionnaie in 8–12-yr-old children. J Behav Ther Exper Ther 2001; 32: 63–72.

Address

Bruce F. Chorpita
Department of Psychology
University of Hawaii at Manoa
2430 Campus Road
Honolulu, HI 96822
USA
chorpita@hawaii.edu

Directions. This form is about worrying. Worrying happens when you are scared about something and you think about it a lot. People sometimes worry about school, their family, their health, things coming up future, or other kinds of things. For each sentence that you read, circle the answer that best tells how true that sentence is about you.

1.	My worries really bother me	never true	sometimes true	most times true	always true
2.	I don't really worry about things	never true	sometimes true	most times true	always true
3.	Many things make me worry	never true	sometimes true	most times true	always true
4.	I know I shouldn't worry about things, but I just can't help it	never true	sometimes true	most times true	always true
5.	When I am under pressure, I worry a lot	never true	sometimes true	most times true	always true
6.	I am always worrying about something	never true	sometimes true	most times true	always true
7.	I find it easy to stop worrying when I want	never true	sometimes true	most times true	always true
8.	When I finish one thing, I start to worry about everything else	never true	sometimes true	most times true	always true
9.	I never worry about anything	never true	sometimes true	most times true	always true
10.	I've been a worrier all my life	never true	sometimes true	most times true	always true
11.	I notice that I have been worrying about things	never true	sometimes true	most times true	always true
12.	Once I start worrying, I can't stop	never true	sometimes true	most times true	always true
13.	I worry all the time	never true	sometimes true	most times true	always true
14.	I worry about things until they are all done	never true	sometimes true	most times true	always true

Physical Arousal Scale for Children (PH-C) and Positive and Negative Affect Schedule for Children (PANAS-C)

Time 15 minutes

Ages 10–18

Time Frame PH-C: last 2 weeks; PANAS-C: last few weeks

Purpose Assessment of positive and negative affect and physiological arousal.

Commentary

The PANAS-C assesses positive and negative affect (Laurent et al., 1999) and the PH-C assesses physical arousal (Laurent et al, 2004). The combination of the two scales assesses all aspects of the tripartite model of emotion.

Versions

The Physical Arousal Scale for Children (PH-C) and Positive and Negative Affect Schedule for Children (PANAS-C) are only available as a self-report form.

Properties

Items PANAS-C comprises 27 items consisting of single words indicating positive and negative affect. The items are rated on a 5-point scale with responses: not much or not much at all, a little, some, quite a lot, a lot. The PH-C has 18 items assessing physical arousal that are rated on a 5-point scale with responses: never, sometimes, about half the time, often, and all the time.

Scales Factor analysis of the items supported the three factors consistent with the tripartite model. The items are scored on three scales which are labeled: Physical Hyperarousal, Positive Affect, and Negative Affect.

Reliability Cronbach's alphas were 0.87 for Physical Hyperarousal in a group of school children, 0.90 and 0.89 for Positive Affect, and 0.94 and 0.92 for Negative Affect in two groups of school children.

Validity Correlations between self-reported anxiety and Physical Hyperarousal were higher than with Negative Affect in a sample of school children. Although the correlation of self-reported depression with Negative Affect was expectedly higher than with Physical Hyperarousal, the difference in the correlations was not significant. Correlations between the Negative Affect scale and self-reported anxiety and depression were high and significant in both a group of school children and a group of clinical children. Furthermore, correlations in these groups between Positive Affect and depression were only moderate as can be expected from the tripartite model, as well as the low correlations between Positive Affect and anxiety. Correlations of the Positive Affect and Negative Affect scales with self-reported anxiety and depression in a group of clinical children were also consistent with the tripartite model.

Norms Means and standard deviations of the Positive Affect and Negative Affect scales are given in Laurent et al. (1999) in a group of 100 school children.

Use No supplementary materials available.

Key references

Chorpita BF, Daleiden EL. Tripartite dimensions of emotion in a clinical sample: measurement strategies and implications for clinical utility. J Consult Clin Psychol 2002; 70: 1150–60.

Laurent J, Catanzaro S, Joiner TE. Development and preliminary validation of the Physiological Hyperarousel scale for Children. Psychol Assess 2004; 16: 373–80.

Laurent J, Catanzaro S, Joiner TE, et al. A measure of positive affect for children: Scale development and preliminary validation. Psychol Assess 1999; 11: 326–38.

Address

Jeff Laurent
1508 Fox Ridge Court
De Pere, WI 54115
USA
Jefflaurent4@yahoo.com

Physical Arousal Scale for Children (PH-C)

How I feel

Please circle the number that best describes how often you have felt or experienced the following during the last two weeks.

Item	Never	Sometimes	About half the time	Often	All the time
Dry mouth	1	2	3	4	5
Sweaty hands/palms	1	2	3	4	5
Tingling (like pins and needles)	1	2	3	4	5
Blushing	1	2	3	4	5
Shaky	1	2	3	4	5
Stomach ache	1	2	3	4	5
Cold flashes/chills	1	2	3	4	5
Dizzy	1	2	3	4	5
Heart pounding	1	2	3	4	5
Sweating when you are not hot	1	2	3	4	5
Can't catch your breath	1	2	3	4	5
Feeling of choking	1	2	3	4	5
Hot flashes	1	2	3	4	5
Numbness (like your foot's asleep)	1	2	3	4	5
Pain in your chest	1	2	3	4	5
Feeling like throwing up	1	2	3	4	5
Tight muscles	1	2	3	4	5
Can't sit still	1	2	3	4	5

Positive and Negative Affect Schedule for Children (PANAS-C)

Feelings and emotions

This scale consists of a number of words that describe different feelings and emotions. Read each item and then circle the appropriate answer next to that word.

Indicate how much you have felt this way during the past few weeks.

Feeling or emotion	Not much or not at all	A little	Some	Quite a bit	A lot
Interested	1	2	3	4	5
Sad	1	2	3	4	5
Frightened	1	2	3	4	5
Alert	1	2	3	4	5
Excited	1	2	3	4	5
Ashamed	1	2	3	4	5
Upset	1	2	3	4	5
Happy	1	2	3	4	5
Strong	1	2	3	4	5
Nervous	1	2	3	4	5
Guilty	1	2	3	4	5
Energetic	1	2	3	4	5
Scared	1	2	3	4	5
Calm	1	2	3	4	5
Miserable	1	2	3	4	5
Jittery	1	2	3	4	5
Cheerful	1	2	3	4	5
Active	1	2	3	4	5
Proud	1	2	3	4	5
Afraid	1	2	3	4	5
Joyful	1	2	3	4	5
Lonely	1	2	3	4	5
Mad	1	2	3	4	5
Fearless	1	2	3	4	5
Disgusted	1	2	3	4	5
Delighted	1	2	3	4	5
Blue	1	2	3	4	5
Daring	1	2	3	4	5
Gloomy	1	2	3	4	5
Lively	1	2	3	4	5

Revised Child Anxiety and Depression Scale (RCADS)

Time 10 minutes

Ages 6–18

Time Frame Not specified

Purpose Assessment of anxiety and depression symptoms corresponding to dimensions of several DSM-IV anxiety disorders and major depression.

Commentary

The RCADS is a revision and extension of the Spence Children's Anxiety Scale (SCAS; Spence, 1998).

Versions

The Revised Child Anxiety and Depression Scale (RCADS) is only available as a self-report form.

Properties

Items The RCADS comprises 47 items which are rated on 4-point scale with responses: never, sometimes, often, and always.

Scales Factor analysis was used to determine the structure of the RCADS. The items are scored on six scales which are labeled according to DSM-IV disorders: Social Phobia, Panic Disorder, Major Depression, Separation Anxiety, Generalized Anxiety, and Obsessive-Compulsive.

Reliability Test–retest correlations across a 1-week interval ranged from 0.65 to 0.80.

Cronbach's alphas ranged from 0.71 to 0.85.

Validity RCADS' Major Depression correlated higher with another self-report of depression than RCADS' anxiety scales. All scales of the RCADS correlated positively with another self-report of anxiety.

The scales of the RCADS discriminated significantly between children with a specific diagnosis and children without a diagnosis, e.g. the scale Social Anxiety discriminated between children with a social phobia diagnosis and children without diagnosis.

Norms A table with means and standard deviations of all scales for 1887 children from the general population can be found in Chorpita et al. (2000) and for 513 clinical children in Chorpita et al. (2005) in which cut-off values for predicting diagnoses are given as well.

Use Scoring instructions are available from Bruce F. Chorpita at the address below.

Key references

Chorpita BF, Moffitt CE, Gray J. Psychometric properties of the Revised Child Anxiety and Depression Scale in a clinical sample. Behav Res Ther 2005; 43: 309–22.

Chorpita BF, Yim L, Moffitt C, Umemoto LA, Francis SE. Assessment of symptoms of DSM-IV anxiety and depression in children: A revised child anxiety and depression scale. Behav Res Ther 2000; 38: 835–55.

Spence SH. A measure of anxiety symptoms among children. Behav Res Ther 1998; 36: 545–66.

Address

Bruce F. Chorpita
Department of Psychology
University of Hawaii at Manoa
2430 Campus Road
Honolulu, HI 96822
USA
chorpita@hawaii.edu

Revised Child Anxiety and Depression Scale (RCADS)

Please put a circle around the word that shows how often each of these things happen to you. There are no right or wrong answers.

1.	I worry about things	Never	Sometimes	Often	Always
2.	I feel sad or empty	Never	Sometimes	Often	Always
3.	When I have a problem, I get a funny feeling in my stomach	Never	Sometimes	Often	Always
4.	I worry when I think I have done poorly at something	Never	Sometimes	Often	Always
5.	I would feel afraid of being on my own at home	Never	Sometimes	Often	Always
6.	Nothing is much fun anymore	Never	Sometimes	Often	Always
7.	I feel scared when I have to take a test	Never	Sometimes	Often	Always
8.	I feel worried when I think someone is angry with me	Never	Sometimes	Often	Always
9.	I worry about being away from my parents	Never	Sometimes	Often	Always
10.	I get bothered by bad or silly thoughts or pictures in my mind	Never	Sometimes	Often	Always
11.	I have trouble sleeping	Never	Sometimes	Often	Always
12.	I worry that I will do badly at my school work	Never	Sometimes	Often	Always
13.	I worry that something awful will happen to someone in my family	Never	Sometimes	Often	Always
14.	I suddenly feel as if I can't breathe when there is no reason for this	Never	Sometimes	Often	Always
15.	I have problems with my appetite	Never	Sometimes	Often	Always
16.	I have to keep checking that I have done things right (like the switch is off, or the door is locked)	Never	Sometimes	Often	Always
17.	I feel scared if I have to sleep on my own	Never	Sometimes	Often	Always
18.	I have trouble going to school in the mornings because I feel nervous or afraid	Never	Sometimes	Often	Always
19.	I have no energy for things	Never	Sometimes	Often	Always
20.	I worry I might look foolish	Never	Sometimes	Often	Always
21.	I am tired a lot	Never	Sometimes	Often	Always
22.	I worry that bad things will happen to me	Never	Sometimes	Often	Always
23.	I can't seem to get bad or silly thoughts out of my head	Never	Sometimes	Often	Always
24.	When I have a problem, my heart beats really fast	Never	Sometimes	Often	Always
25.	I cannot think clearly	Never	Sometimes	Often	Always
26.	I suddenly start to tremble or shake when there is no reason for this	Never	Sometimes	Often	Always
27.	I worry that something bad will happen to me	Never	Sometimes	Often	Always
28.	When I have a problem, I feel shaky	Never	Sometimes	Often	Always
29.	I feel worthless	Never	Sometimes	Often	Always
30.	I worry about making mistakes	Never	Sometimes	Often	Always
31.	I have to think of special thoughts (like numbers or words) to stop bad things from happening	Never	Sometimes	Often	Always
32.	I worry what other people think of me	Never	Sometimes	Often	Always
33.	I am afraid of being in crowded places (like shopping centers, the movies, buses, busy playgrounds)	Never	Sometimes	Often	Always
34.	All of a sudden I feel really scared for no reason at all	Never	Sometimes	Often	Always
35.	I worry about what is going to happen	Never	Sometimes	Often	Always
36.	I suddenly become dizzy or faint when there is no reason for this	Never	Sometimes	Often	Always
37.	I think about death	Never	Sometimes	Often	Always
38.	I feel afraid if I have to talk in front of my class	Never	Sometimes	Often	Always
39.	My heart suddenly starts to beat too quickly for no reason	Never	Sometimes	Often	Always
40.	I feel like I don't want to move	Never	Sometimes	Often	Always
41.	I worry that I will suddenly get a scared feeling when there is nothing to be afraid of	Never	Sometimes	Often	Always
42.	I have to do some things over and over again (like washing my hands, cleaning or putting things in a certain order)	Never	Sometimes	Often	Always
43.	I feel afraid that I will make a fool of myself in front of people	Never	Sometimes	Often	Always
44.	I have to do some things in just the right way to stop bad things from happening	Never	Sometimes	Often	Always
45.	I worry when I go to bed at night	Never	Sometimes	Often	Always
46.	I would feel scared if I had to stay away from home overnight	Never	Sometimes	Often	Always
47.	I feel restless	Never	Sometimes	Often	Always

Revised Children's Manifest Anxiety Scale (RCMAS)

Time 5–10 minutes

Ages 6–19

Time Frame Not specified

Purpose Assessment of anxiety problems.

Commentary

The RCMAS, subtitled 'What I Think and Feel,' is a revision of the Children's Manifest Anxiety Scale (CMAS; Castaneda et al, 1956), and the CMAS was adapted from a scale for adults first reported in 1951. In routine psychoeducational assessment of children, a measure of anxiety should be included. The RCMAS is such a measure that provides indications of multiple aspects of anxiety.

Versions

The Revised Children's Manifest Anxiety Scale (RCMAS) is only available as a self-report form.

Properties

Items The RCMAS comprises 28 items assessing anxiety and 9 items indicating response bias. All items are rated on a 2-point scale with responses: yes and no.

Scales Factor analysis was used to investigate the scale structure. The 28 anxiety items are scored on three scales labeled Physiological Anxiety, Worry/Oversensitivity, and Social Concerns/Concentration. The 28 items also constitute the Total Anxiety Score. The nine items indicating response bias form the Lie subscale.

Reliability Cronbach's alphas were 0.67 for Physiological Anxiety, 0.76 for Worry/Oversensitivity, 0.64 for Social Concerns/Concentration, 0.84 for Total Anxiety, and 0.77 for the Lie subscale.

Validity The RCMAS scales correlated highly with trait anxiety symptoms and did not correlate with state anxiety symptoms.

Norms The RCMAS was standardized on a sample of 4972 children from the general population. For interpretation purposes raw scores were converted to percentiles and scaled scores.

Use A manual and forms can be obtained from the publisher at the address below. A table that lists all items can be found in Reynolds and Richmond (1978).

Key references

Castaneda A, McCandless BR, Palermo DS. The children's form of the manifest anxiety scale. Child Dev 1956; 27: 317–26.

Reynolds CR, Richmond BO. What I think and feel: A revised measure of children's manifest anxiety. J Abnorm Child Psychol 1978; 6: 271–80.

Reynolds CR, Richmond BO. Revised Children's Manifest Anxiety Scale: Manual. Los Angeles: Western Psychological Services, 1985.

Address

Western Psychological Services
12031 Wilshire Blvd.
Los Angeles, CA 90025–1251
USA
www.wpspublish.com

Revised Children's Manifest Anxiety Scale (RCMAS) – sample items

Yes No	1.	I have trouble making up my mind.	
Yes No	5.	Often I have trouble getting my breath.	
Yes No	10.	I worry about what my parents will say to me.	
Yes No	18.	My feelings get hurt easily.	

Yes No	23.	Other people are happier than I.
Yes No	27.	I feel someone will tell me I do things the wrong way.
Yes No	32.	I never say things I shouldn't.
Yes No	36.	I never lie.

Screen for Child Anxiety Related Emotional Disorders (SCARED)

Time 10–15 minutes

Ages 6–18

Time Frame Last 3 months, but can be used as a current or lifetime instrument

Purpose Assessment of anxiety symptoms.

Commentary

The SCARED was developed because available self-report instruments did not differentiate between individual anxiety disorders. Therefore, the SCARED was conceived as a practical screening instrument for the assessment of general anxiety disorder, separation anxiety disorder, panic disorder, social phobia, and school phobia.

Versions

The Screen for Child Anxiety Related Emotional Disorders (SCARED) is available as a parent report for ages 6–18 years and as a self-report for ages 8–18. Clinicians can read the questions to children aged 6 and 7 years.

Properties

Items   The SCARED comprises 41 items that are rated on a 3-point scale with responses: not true or hardly ever true, somewhat true or sometimes true, and very true or often true.

Scales   Factor analysis supported five factors. Therefore, the items of the SCARED are scored on five subscales with labels: panic/somatic, general anxiety, separation anxiety, social phobia, and school phobia. In addition, the total anxiety score is the simple sum of all items.

Reliability   Test–retest intraclass correlations a cross a median 5-week interval ranged from 0.70 to 0.90 for the five subscales and was 0.86 for the total score.

Cronbach's alphas ranged from 0.74 to 0.89 for the subscales and it was 0.90 for the total score.

Validity   The parent-reported total score correlated significantly higher with parent-reported internalizing problems than with externalizing problems. The five subscales correlated significantly with subscales of parent-reported internalizing problems, but did not correlate with externalizing problems. Parent- and child-reported total score and the subscale scores correlated significantly with parent- and self-reported trait and state anxiety scores. However, the correlations with trait anxiety were significantly higher than with state anxiety.

Mean scores of the SCARED total scale and subscales were significantly higher for children diagnosed with anxiety disorders than for children diagnosed with other disorders. Furthermore, mean scores for the self-report form were significantly higher for children diagnosed with anxiety disorders than for children diagnosed with depressive disorders. However, these differences were only significant for the total score, panic/somatic score, and separation anxiety for the parent form. Total score and subscale scores of both self-report and parent form were significantly higher for children diagnosed with anxiety disorders than for children diagnosed with disruptive disorders, except for self-reported separation anxiety and parent-reported social phobia. The child and parent SCARED significantly discriminated anxiety from other disorders, with one exception: the parent SCARED did not significantly discriminate between anxiety and depression. The SCARED has been validated in clinical as well as community samples in different countries. The SCARED is sensitive to treatment effects.

Norms   A cut-off value of 25 on the child SCARED total score was determined as the optimum point for discriminating between anxiety and non-anxiety, anxiety and depression, and anxiety and disruptive disorders with sensitivity of 71% and specificity of 67%, 61%, and 71%, respectively. Some children may have significant anxiety symptoms in one of more factors, but the total score can be below 25. Thus, it is recommended that in addition to the total score, symptoms for each factor will be added separately.

Use   The rating scales and instructions can be downloaded at the website below, under 'Research' and then 'Assessment Instruments'.

Key references

Birmaher B, Brent DA, Chiappetta L, et al. Psychometric properties of the Screen for Child Anxiety Related Emotional Disorders (SCARED): A replication study. J Am Acad Child Adolesc Psychiatry 1999; 38: 1230–6.

Birmaher B, Khetarpai S, Brent D, et al. The Screen of Child Anxiety Related Emotional Disorders (SCARED): Scale construction and psychometric characteristics. J Am Acad Child Adolesc Psychiatry 1997; 36: 545–53.

Monga S, Birmaher B, Chiappetta L, et al. Screen for Child Anxiety-Related Emotional Disorders (SCARED): Convergent and divergent validity. Depress Anx 2000; 12: 85–91.

Address

Boris Birmaher
Department of Child Psychiatry
University of Pittsburgh Medical Center
Western Psychiatric Institute and Clinic
Pittsburgh PA 15213
USA
birmaherb@upmc.edu
www.wpic.pitt-edu

Screen for Child Anxiety Related Emotional Disorders (SCARED) – Parent Version

(To be filled out by the parent)

Name: _____   Date: _____

Directions: Below is a list of statements that describe how people feel. Read each statement carefully and decide if it is 'not true or hardly ever true' or 'somewhat true or sometimes true' or 'very true of often true' for your child. Then for each statement, fill in one circle that corresponds to the response that seems to describe your child *for the last 3 months*. Please respond to all statements as well as you can, even if some do not seem to concern your child.

	0 Not true or hardly ever true	1 Somewhat true or sometimes true	2 Very true or often true
1. When my child feels frightened, it is hard for him/her to breathe	○	○	○
2. My child gets headaches when he/she is at school	○	○	○
3. My child doesn't like to be with people he/she doesn't know well	○	○	○
4. My child gets scared if he/she sleeps away from home	○	○	○
5. My child worries about other people liking him/her	○	○	○
6. When my child gets frightened, he/she feels like passing out	○	○	○
7. My child is nervous	○	○	○
8. My child follows me wherever I go	○	○	○
9. People tell me that my child looks nervous	○	○	○
10. My child feels nervous with people he/she doesn't know well	○	○	○
11. My child gets stomach aches at school	○	○	○
12. When my child gets frightened, he/she feels like he/she is going crazy	○	○	○
13. My child worries about sleeping alone	○	○	○
14. My child worries about being as good as other kids	○	○	○
15. When he/she gets frightened, he/she feels like things are not real	○	○	○
16. My child has nightmares about something bad happening to his/her parents	○	○	○
17. My child worries about going to school	○	○	○
18. When my child gets frightened, his/her heart beats fast	○	○	○
19. He/she gets shaky	○	○	○
20. My child has nightmares about something bad happening to him/her	○	○	○
21. My child worries about things working out for him/her	○	○	○
22. When my child gets frightened, he/she sweats a lot	○	○	○
23. My child is a worrier	○	○	○
24. My child gets really frightened for no reason at all	○	○	○
25. My child is afraid to be alone in the house	○	○	○
26. It is hard for my child to talk to people he/she doesn't know well	○	○	○
27. When my child gets frightened, he/she feels like he/she is choking	○	○	○
28. People tell me that my child worries too much	○	○	○
29. My child doesn't like to be away from his/her family	○	○	○
30. My child is afraid of having anxiety (or panic) attacks	○	○	○
31. My child worries that something bad might happen to his/her parents	○	○	○
32. My child feels shy with people he/she doesn't know well	○	○	○
33. My child worries about what is going to happen in the future	○	○	○
34. When my child gets frightened, he/she feels like throwing up	○	○	○
35. My child worries about how well he/she does things	○	○	○
36. My child is scared to go to school	○	○	○
37. My child worries about things that have already happened	○	○	○
38. When my child gets frightened, he/she feels dizzy	○	○	○
39. My child feels nervous when he/she is with other children or adults and he/she has to do something while they watch him/her (for example: read aloud, speak, play a game, play a sport)	○	○	○
40. My child feels nervous when he/she is going to parties, dances, or any place where there will be people that he/she doesn't know	○	○	○
41. My child is shy	○	○	○

Screen for Child Anxiety Related Emotional Disorders (SCARED) – Child Version

(To be filled out by the child)

Name: _____   Date: _____

Directions*: Below is a list of sentences that describe how people feel. Read each phrase and decide if it is 'not true or hardly ever true' or 'somewhat true or sometimes true' or 'very true or often true' for you. Then for each sentence, fill in one circle that corresponds to the response that seems to describe you for *the last 3 months*.

		0 Not true or hardly ever true	1 Somewhat true or sometimes true	2 Very true or often true
1.	When I feel frightened, it is hard to breathe	○	○	○
2.	I get headaches when I am at school	○	○	○
3.	I don't like to be with people I don't know well	○	○	○
4.	I get scared if I sleep away from home	○	○	○
5.	I worry about other people liking me	○	○	○
6.	When I get frightened, I feel like passing out	○	○	○
7.	I am nervous	○	○	○
8.	I follow my mother or father wherever they go	○	○	○
9.	People tell me that I look nervous	○	○	○
10.	I feel nervous with people I don't know well	○	○	○
11.	I get stomach aches at school	○	○	○
12.	When I get frightened, I feel like I am going crazy	○	○	○
13.	I worry about sleeping alone	○	○	○
14.	I worry about being as good as other kids	○	○	○
15.	When I get frightened, I feel like things are not real	○	○	○
16.	I have nightmares about something bad happening to my parents	○	○	○
17.	I worry about going to school	○	○	○
18.	When I get frightened, my heart beats fast	○	○	○
19.	I get shaky	○	○	○
20.	I have nightmares about something bad happening to me	○	○	○
21.	I worry about things working out for me	○	○	○
22.	When I get frightened, I sweat a lot	○	○	○
23.	I am a worrier	○	○	○
24.	I get really frightened for no reason at all	○	○	○
25.	I am afraid to be alone in the house	○	○	○
26.	It is hard for me to talk with people I don't know well	○	○	○
27.	When I get frightened, I feel like I am choking	○	○	○
28.	People tell me that I worry too much	○	○	○
29.	I don't like to be away from my family	○	○	○
30.	I am afraid of having anxiety (or panic) attacks	○	○	○
31.	I worry that something bad might happen to my parents	○	○	○
32.	I feel shy with people I don't know well	○	○	○
33.	I worry about what is going to happen in the future	○	○	○
34.	When I get frightened, I feel like throwing up	○	○	○
35.	I worry about how well I do things	○	○	○
36.	I am scared to go to school	○	○	○
37.	I worry about things that have already happened	○	○	○
38.	When I get frightened, I get dizzy	○	○	○
39.	I feel nevous when I am with other children or adults and I have to do something while they watch me (for example: read aloud, speak, play a game, play a sport)	○	○	○
40.	I feel nervous when I am going to parties, dances, or any place where there will be people that I don't know well	○	○	○
41.	I am shy	○	○	○

Scoring

A total score of ≥25 may indicate the presence of an **anxiety disorder**. Scores higher than 30 are more specific. A score of 7 for items 1, 6, 9, 12, 15, 18, 19, 22, 24, 27, 30, 34, 38 may indicate **panic disorder** or **significant somatic symptoms**.

A score of 9 for items 5, 7, 14, 21, 23, 28, 33, 35, 37 may indicate **generalized anxiety disorder**.

A score of 5 for items 4, 8, 13, 16, 20, 25, 29, 31 may indicate **separation anxiety disorder**.

A score of 8 for items 3, 10, 26, 32, 39, 40, 41 may indicate **social anxiety disorder**.

A score of 3 for items 2, 11, 17, 36 may indicate **significant school avoidance**.

*For children aged 8–11, it is recommended that the clinician explain all questions, or have the child answer the questionnaire sitting with an adult in case they have any questions.

© Boris Birmaher. Reproduced by permission.

Social Anxiety Scale for Children-Revised (SASC-R) and Social Anxiety Scale for Adolescents (SAS-A)

Time 10 minutes

Ages SASC-R: 6–13; SAS-A: 13–18

Time Frame Not specified

Purpose Assessment of social anxiety problems.

Commentary

The SASC-R was adapted from the SASC that first appeared in 1988 (La Greca et al, 1988). The SAS-A was adapted from the SASC-R. The wording of the SAS-A was made more age appropriate for adolescents.

Versions

The Social Anxiety Scale for Children-Revised (SASC-R) and Social Anxiety Scale for Adolescents (SAS-A) are both available as parent reports and self-reports.

Properties

Items Both the SASR-C and SAS-A comprise 22 items of which 18 pertain to social anxiety and four are filler items. The items are rated on a 5-point scale with responses from not at all to all the time.

Scales The items of both scales can be scored on three subscales, which were supported by factor analysis. The three subscales are: Fear of Negative Evaluation (FNE) reflecting fears for negative evaluations from peers, SAD-New reflecting social avoidance and distress with new social situations, and SAD-General reflecting generalized social distress.

Reliability Cronbach's alphas for the SASC-R subscales FNE, SAD-New, and SAD-General were 0.86, 0.78, and 0.69, respectively in a sample of school children, and 0.90, 0.74, 0.60, respectively in a sample of clinical children. For the SAS-A subscales FNE, SAD-New, and SAD-General, Cronbach's alphas were 0.91, 0.83, and 0.76, respectively in a sample of high school students.

Validity Correlations of the SASC-R subscales with self-perceptions of social acceptance, global self-worth, and behavioral conduct ranged from –0.12 to –0.47.

Correlations were highest between social anxiety and social acceptance and lowest between social anxiety and behavioral conduct.

Median correlations of the SAS-A subscales FNE, SAD-New, and SAD-General were with peer relations variables –0.45, –0.48, and –0.41 for girls, and –0.24, –0.24, .and –0.28 for boys, with close friendship variables –0.29, –0.44, and –0.29 for girls, and –0.09, –0.13, and –0.14 for boys, and with non-peer-related support variables –0.11, –0.18, –0.15 for girls, and –0.08, –0.05, and –0.12 for boys.

Clinical children with a comorbid social anxiety disorder had significantly higher scores on all SASC-R subscales than those without a comorbid social anxiety disorder.

To investigate associations between social anxiety assessed with the SASC-R and peer status, children were classified into four social-status groups: popular, rejected, neglected, and average. For the FNE subscale, children in rejected and neglected groups had significantly higher scores than children in popular and average groups, but the rejected and neglected groups did not differ from each other. For the SAD-New and SAD-General subscales, children in the neglected group had higher scores than children in the three other groups, and those in the rejected group had higher scores than children in the popular and average groups.

Norms A table with means and standard deviations of the SASC-R subscales for 459 schoolchildren aged 9–13 separated by sex and grade is printed in La Greca and Stone (1993). A table with means and standard deviations of the SAS-A subscales for 250 high school students aged 15–18 years separated by sex is printed in La Greca and Lopez (1998). Additional normative data for the SAS-A can be found in Inderbitzen-Nolan and Walter (2000) and Storch et al (2004).

Use The SASC-R, SAS-A and a manual describing both scales can be obtained from Annette M. La Greca at the address below.

Key references

Inderbitzen-Nolan HM, Walters KS. Social Anxiety Scale for Adolescents: Normative data and further evidence of construct validity. J Clin Child Psychol 2000; 29: 360–71.

Ginsburg GS, La Greca AM, Silverman WK. Social anxiety in children with anxiety disorders: Relation with social and emotional functioning. J Abnorm Child Psychol 1998; 26: 175–85.

La Greca AM, Dandes SK, Wick P, Shaw K, Stone WL. Development of the Social Anxiety Scale for Children: Reliability and concurrent validity. J Clin Child Psychol 1988; 17: 84–91.

La Greca AM, Lopez N. Social anxiety among adolescents: Linkages with peer relations and friendships. J Abnorm Child Psychol 1998; 26: 83–94.

La Greca AM, Stone WL. Social Anxiety Scale for Children-Revised: Factor structure and concurrent validity. J Clin Child Psychol 1993; 22: 17–27.

Storch EA, Masia-Warner C, Dent HC, Roberti JW, Fisher PH. Psychometric evaluation of the Social Anxiety Scale for Adolescents and the Social Phobia and Anxiety Inventory for children: Construct validity and normative data. J Anxiety Dis 2004; 18: 665–79.

Address

Annette M. La Greca
Department of Psychology
P.O. Box 249229
Coral Gables, Florida 33124
USA
alagreca@miami.edu

Social Phobia and Anxiety Inventory for Children (SPAI-C)

Time 20–30 minutes

Ages 8–14

Time Frame Not specified

Purpose Assessment of social anxiety problems.

Commentary

The development of the SPAI-C was motivated by the fact that a large number of children coming to a specialty clinic met criteria for social phobia.

Versions

The Social Phobia and Anxiety Inventory for Children (SPAI-C) is only available as a self-report.

Properties

Items   The SPAI-C comprises 26 items of which 16 consist of three to five items, so that the total number of items that have to be rated is 63. All items are rated on a 3-point scale with responses: never, or hardly ever; sometimes; and most of the time, or always.

Scales   The items of the SPAI-C are scored on the Total Score which is the simple sum of all item ratings. Factor analysis also supported subscales, but the constellation of subscales depended on characteristics of respondents. Three to five factors were found, including assertiveness, general conversation, and public performance.

Reliability   Test–retest correlation for the Total Score was 0.86 across a 2-week interval and 0.63 across a 10-month interval in a group of children with predominantly anxiety disorders.

Cronbach's alpha was 0.95 in a group of children with predominantly anxiety disorders and 0.92 in a group of children with social phobia, externalizing disorder, or no disorder.

Validity   Correlations of the Total Score with self-reported phobic fears ranged from 0.41 to 0.53. The correlation with fear of failure and criticism was the highest. Correlations of the Total Score with trait and state anxiety were 0.50 and 0.13, respectively. Correlations of the Total Score with mother-reported internalizing and externalizing problems were 0.45 and 0.18, respectively and with social competence –0.33. The Total Score correlated 0.50 with the number of daily social events and 0.41 with the distress these events incurred.

Discriminant analysis was to determine how well the Total Score could distinguish children with social phobia and children with other disorders. The Total Score discriminated between the groups with a sensitivity of 70% and a specificity of 80%. The Total Score was significantly higher in a group of children with social phobia than in a group of children with externalizing disorder and than in a group of children with no disorder. In a comparison of children with social phobia and children with other anxiety disorders, the children with social phobia had significantly higher scores on the Total Score.

Norms   Cut-off scores were determined in a combined sample of 52 children with anxiety disorder and 48 controls aged 8–17 years. Further normative data on 1178 high school students aged 13–17 years can be found in Storch et al (2004).

Use   A manual and rating scales enabling direct scoring are available from the publisher at the address below.

Key references

Beidel DC, Turner MS, Morris TL. SPAI-C Social Phobia & Anxiety Inventory for Children. North Tonawanda, NY: Multi-Health Systems Inc, 1998.

Beidel DC, Turner MS, Morris TL. A new inventory to assess childhood social anxiety and phobia: The Social Phobia and Anxiety Inventory for Children. Psychol Assess 1995; 7: 73–9.

Storch EA, Masia-Warner C, Dent HC, Roberti JW, Fisher PH. Psychometric evaluation of the Social Anxiety Scale for Adolescents and the Social Phobia and Anxiety Inventory for children: Construct validity and normative data. J Anxiety Disord 2004; 18: 665–79.

Address

Multi-Health Systems Inc.
P.O. Box 950
North Tonawanda, NY 14120–0950
USA
www.mhs.com

Social Phobia and Anxiety Inventory for Children (SPAI-C) – sample items

		Never, or hardly ever	Sometimes	Most of the time, or always
4.	I feel scared when I have to speak or read in front of a group of people	0	1	2
8.	I am too scared to ask questions in class	0	1	2
14.	I feel scared when I start to talk to			
	boys or girls my age that I know	0	1	2
	boys or girls my age that I don't know	0	1	2
	adults	0	1	2
18.	I feel scared when I am ignored or made fun of by			
	boys or girls my age that I know	0	1	2
	boys or girls my age that I don't know	0	1	2
	adults	0	1	2
24.	When I am with other people, I think scary thoughts. Sometimes I think			
	if I goof up, I will really feel bad	0	1	2
	what are they thinking of me?	0	1	2
	whatever I say will sound stupid	0	1	2

Spence Children's Anxiety Scale (SCAS)

Time 5–10 minutes

Ages 7–19

Time Frame Not specified

Purpose Assessment of anxiety symptoms consistent with DSM-IV classification.

Commentary

The SCAS is a recent development, but is already translated in several languages and used in several studies. The website provides information about its use, psychometric properties and English forms and papers for download.

Versions

The Spence Children's Anxiety Scale (SCAS) comprises self-report and parent-report forms. A version for preschoolers is also available.

Properties

Items The SCAS comprises 45 items, of which 38 reflect specific anxiety symptoms, one open-ended question, and six are positive filler items. All items are scored on a 4-point scale with responses: never, sometimes, often, and always.

Scales The results of confirmatory factor analyses of children's responses from community samples supported six factors consistent with hypothesized diagnostic categories. Scale names are: Panic/Agoraphobia, Separation Anxiety, Social Phobia, Physical Injury Fears, Obsessive-compulsive Disorder, and Generalized Anxiety Disorder/Overanxious Disorder.

Reliability Correlations over a 12-week interval were between 0.53 and 0.69 and over a 6-month interval between 0.45 and 0.60.

Most Cronbach's alphas were in the 0.70–0.80 range, but for Fear of Physical Injury 0.60 or lower and for the Total Score 0.90 or higher.

Validity The SCAS correlated 0.71 and 0.89 with other anxiety measures. The SCAS correlated 0.48 with depression, but this correlation was significantly lower than the correlation with the RCMAS. Referred children had significantly higher anxiety scores than control children.

Norms The website lists means, standard deviations, and cut-off values for various samples taken from published papers.

Use Information about use and properties can be found available on the website at the address below, where rating scales can be downloaded as well.

Key references

Spence SH. Structure of anxiety symptoms among children: A confirmatory factor-analytic study. J Abnorm Psychol 1997; 106: 280–97.

Spence SH. A measure of anxiety symptoms among children. Behav Res Ther 1998; 36: 545–66.

Spence SH, Barrett PM, Turner CM. Psychometric properties of the Spence Children's Anxiety Scale with young adolescents. J Anxiety Disord 2003; 17: 605–25.

Address

Susan H. Spence
Department of Psychology
University of Queensland
Brisbane
QLD 4072
Australia
s.spence@psy.uq.edu.au
www2.psy.uq.edu.au/~sues/scas

State-Trait Anxiety Inventory for Children (STAIC)

Time 20 minutes

Ages Grades 4–6

Time Frame State anxiety items: now; Trait anxiety items: usually

Purpose Assessment of state and trait anxiety.

Commentary

The STAIC is based on the State-Trait Anxiety Inventory for adults (Spielberger et al. 1970).

Versions

The State-Trait Anxiety Inventory for Children (STAIC) is available in only a self-report form.

Properties

Items   The STAIC comprises 20 items assessing state anxiety and 20 items assessing trait anxiety. The state anxiety items all start with the stem 'I feel' and next to each stem are three responses from which respondents has to pick one that best describes their state, for example: very calm, calm, and not calm. The trait anxiety items are rated on a 4-point scale with responses: hardly-ever, sometimes, and often.

Scales   The state anxiety items are scored on the S-Anxiety scale, and the trait anxiety items are scored on the T-Anxiety scale.

Reliability   Test–retest correlations across a 6-week interval were for S-Anxiety 0.31 for boys and 0.47 for girls, and were for T-Anxiety 0.65 for boys and 0.71 for girls.

Cronbach's alphas were for S-Anxiety 0.82 for boys and 0.87 for girls, and were for T-Anxiety 0.78 for boys and 0.81 for girls.

Validity   The T-Anxiety scale correlated high with other self-reports of trait anxiety.

Children reported higher S-Anxiety scores when they are in a stressful condition than in a normal condition.

Norms   The STAIC was standardized on 1551 elementary school children in grades 4 to 6. Raw scores were converted to normalized T-scores and percentiles. Tables containing norms are presented in Spielberger (1973) as well as tables with means and standard deviations.

Use   A manual and rating forms can be obtained from the publisher at the address below. The manual contains a bibliography updated in 1997 which lists research conducted with the STAIC. The STAIC is translated in several languages.

Key references

Spielberger CD. State-Trait Anxiety Inventory for Children – STAIC: Professional Manual. Redwood City: Mind Garden, Inc, 1973.

Spielberger CD, Gorsuch RL, Lushene RE. Manual for the State-Trait Anxiety Inventory (Self-Evaluation Questionnaire). Palo Alto: Consulting Psychologists Press, 1970.

Address

Mind Garden, Inc.
1690 Woodside Road, Suite 202
Redwood City
California 94061
USA
www.mindgarden.com

3.2 Obsessive Compulsive Disorders

Children's Obsessional Compulsive Inventory (CHOCI)

Time 15 minutes

Ages 7–17

Time Frame Not specified

Purpose Assessment of obsessive and compulsive problems.

Commentary

The CHOCI was developed for the assessment of content and severity of obsessive and compulsive symptoms. It was designed as a self-report as opposed to the time-consuming clinician-rated CY-BOCS which is described below.

Versions

The Children's Obsessional Compulsive Inventory (CHOCI) is only available as a self-report form.

Properties

Items The CHOCI comprises two parts: the first part has items pertaining to compulsive problems and the second part has items pertaining to obsessive problems. Each part comprises ten items representing symptoms and five items representing impairment ratings of the symptoms. The symptom items are rated on a 3-point scale with responses: not at all, somewhat, and a lot. The impairment ratings are rated on a 5-point scale with responses from not impaired to very impaired, but the responses are not identical for all items.

Scales The items of the CHOCI are scored on four subscales which are labeled: Obsessions symptom, Obsessions impairment, Compulsions symptoms, and Compulsions impairment. In addition, the sum of both impairment subscales constitutes the Total impairment scale.

Reliability Cronbach's alphas were above 0.80 for all four subscales.

Validity The CHOCI impairment subscales and Total impairment correlated 0.38, 0.42, and 0.49 with clinician-reported obsessive and compulsive symptoms.

Means for all scales were significantly different between children diagnosed with an obsessive compulsive disorder and children with no known disorders.

Norms No information available.

Use No supplemental information available.

Key references

Shafran R, Frampton I, Heyman I, et al. The preliminary development of a new self-report measure for OCD in young people. J Adolesc 2003; 26: 137–42.

Address

Roz Shafran
Oxford University Department of Psychiatry
Warnefond Hospital
Oxford OX3 7JX
United Kingdom
roz.shafran@psych.ox.ac.uk

To be completed by the young person

Date: _____ Age: _____ Sex: Male/Female

ChOCI: Part I

Each of the following questions asks you about things or 'habits' you feel you have to do although you may know that they do not make sense. Sometimes, you may try to stop from doing them but this might not be possible. You might feel worried or angry or frustrated until you have finished what you have to do. An example of a habit like this may be the need to wash your hands over and over again even though they are not really dirty, or the need to count up to a special number (e.g., 6 or 10) while you do certain things.

 Please answer each question by putting a circle around the number that best describes how much you agree with the statement, or how much you think it is true of you. Please answer each item, without spending too much time on any one item. There are no right or wrong answers.

Example:	**Not at all**	**Somewhat**	**A lot**
I feel that I must check and check again that the stove is turned off, even if I don't want to do so.	1	2	3

How much do you agree with each of the following statements?	**Not at all**	**Somewhat**	**A lot**
1. I spend far too much time washing my hands over and over again.	1	2	3
2. I feel I must do ordinary/everyday things exactly the same way, every time I do them.	1	2	3
3. I spend a lot of time every day checking things over and over and over again.	1	2	3
4. I often have trouble finishing things because I need to make absolutely sure that everything is exactly right.	1	2	3
5. I spend far too much time arranging my things in order.	1	2	3
6. I need someone to tell me things are alright over and over again.	1	2	3
7. If I touch something with one hand, I feel I absolutely must touch the same thing with the other hand, in order to make things even and equal.	1	2	3
8. I always count, even when doing ordinary things.	1	2	3
9. If I have a 'bad thought', I always have to make sure that I immediately have a 'good thought' to cancel it out	1	2	3
10. I am often very late because I keep on repeating the same action, over and over again.	1	2	3

Please try to think about the three *most* upsetting **habits** that you feel you **have** to do and **can't stop**. For example, feeling that you have to wash your hands far too often, or repeating the same action over and over, or constantly checking that the doors and windows are shut properly.

1) _____

2) _____

3) _____

How much time do you spend doing these habits? Please circle the answer that best describes you.

0	1	2	3	4
None	Less than 1 hr. a day (occasionally)	1-3 hrs. a day (part of a morning or afternoon)	3-8 hrs. a day (about half the time you're awake)	More than 8 hrs. a day (almost all the time you're awake)

How much do these habits get in the way of school or doing things with friends? Please circle the answer that best describes you.

0	1	2	3	4
Not at all	A little	Somewhat	A lot	Almost always

How would you feel if prevented from carrying out your habits? How upset would you become? Please circle the answer that best describes you.

0	1	2	3	4
Not at all	A little	Somewhat	A lot	Totally

How much do you try to fight the upsetting habits? Please circle the answer that best describes you.

0	1	2	3	4
I always try to resist	I try to resist most of the time	I make some effort to resist	Even though I want to, I don't try to resist	I don't resist at all

How strong is the feeling that you have to carry out the habits? Please circle the answer that best describes you.

0	1	2	3	4
Not strong	Mild pressure to carry out habits	Strong pressure to carry out habits; hard to control	Very strong pressure to carry out habits; very hard to control	Extreme pressure to carry out habits; impossible to control

How much have you been avoiding doing anything, going any place, or being with anyone because of your upsetting habits? Please circle the answer that best describes you.

0	1	2	3	4
Not at all	A little	Somewhat	A lot	Almost always

ChOCI: Part 2

In this section, each of the questions asks you about *thoughts, ideas, or pictures* that keep coming into your mind even though you do not want them to do so. They may be unpleasant, silly, or embarrassing. For example, some young people have the repeated thought that germs or dirt are harming them or other people, or that something unpleasant may happen to them or someone special to them. **These are thoughts that keep coming back, over and over again, even though you do not want them.**

Please answer each question by putting a circle around the number that best describes how much you agree with the statement, or how much you think it is true of you. Please answer each item, without spending too much time on any one item. There are no right or wrong answers.

Example: I often have the same upsetting thought about death over and over again.	Not at all 1	Somewhat 2	A lot 3

How much do you agree with each of the following statements?	Not at all	Somewhat	A lot
1. I can't stop thinking upsetting thoughts about an accident.	1	2	3
2. I often have bad thoughts that make me feel like a terrible person.	1	2	3
3. Upsetting thoughts about my family being hurt go round and round in my head and stop me from concentrating.	1	2	3
4. I always have big doubts about whether I've made the right decision, even about stupid little things	1	2	3
5. I can't stop upsetting thoughts about death from going round in my head, over and over again.	1	2	3
6. I often have mean thoughts about other people that I feel are terrible, over and over again.	1	2	3
7. I often have horrible thoughts about going crazy.	1	2	3
8. I keep on having frightening thoughts that something terrible is going to happen and it will be my fault.	1	2	3
9. I'm very frightened that I will think something (or do something) that will upset God	1	2	3
10. I'm always worried that my mean thoughts about other people are as wicked as actually doing mean things to them	1	2	3

Please list the three most severe **thoughts** that you often have **and can't stop thinking about**. For example, thinking about hurting someone, or thinking bad things about God.

1) _____

2) _____

3) _____

How much time do you spend thinking about these things? Please circle the answer that best describes you.

0	1	2	3	4
None	Less than 1 hr. a day (occasionally)	1-3 hrs. a day (part of a morning or afternoon)	3-8 hrs. a day (about half the time you're awake)	More than 8 hrs. a day (almost all the time you're awake)

How much do these thoughts get in the way of school or doing things with friends? Please circle the answer that best describes you.

0	1	2	3	4
Not at all	A little	Somewhat	A lot	Extreme

How much do these thoughts bother or upset you? Please circle the answer that best describes you.

0	1	2	3	4
Not at all	A little	Somewhat	A lot	Extreme

How hard do you try to stop the thoughts or ignore them? Please circle the answer that best describes you.

0	1	2	3	4
I always try to resist	I try to resist most of the time	I make some effort to resist	Even though I want to, I don't try to resist	I don't resist at all

When you try to fight the thoughts, can you beat them? How much control do you have over the thoughts? Please circle the answer that best describes you.

0	1	2	3	4
Complete control	Much control	Moderate control	Little control	No control

How much have you been avoiding doing anything, going any place, or being with anyone because of your thoughts? Please circle the answer that best describes you.

0	1	2	3	4
Not at all	A little	Somewhat	A lot	Almost always

To be completed by the child/adolescent

CHOCI: Part I

Each of the following questions asks you about things or 'habits' you feel you have to do although you may know that they do not make sense. Sometimes, you may try to stop from doing them but this might not be possible. You might feel worried or angry or frustrated until you have finished what you have to do. An example of a habit like this may be the need to wash your hands over and over again even though they are not really dirty, or the need to count up to a special number (e.g., 6 or 10) while you do certain things.

Please answer each question by putting a circle around the number that best describes how much you agree with the statement, or how much you think it is true of you. Please answer each item, without spending too much time on any one item. There are no right or wrong answers.

Example:	**Not at all**	**Somewhat**	**A lot**
I feel that I must check and check again that the stove is turned off, even if I don't want to do so.	1	2	3

How much do you agree with each of the following statements?	**Not at all**	**Somewhat**	**A lot**
1. I spend far too much time washing my hands over and over again.	1	2	3
2. I feel I must check my homework over and over and over again.	1	2	3
3. I feel I must do ordinary/everyday things exactly the same way, every time I do them.	1	2	3
4. I find it very difficult to throw things away so my room is much too crowded/cluttered.	1	2	3
5. I am too scared to use public toilets because of dirt/germs.	1	2	3
6. I check and check things like taps and switches over and over again.	1	2	3
7. I get really upset if my things are not always in exactly the same place.	1	2	3
8. I often get behind in my school work because I write the same words over and over and over again.	1	2	3
9. I am much, much too concerned about being clean.	1	2	3
10. I spend a lot of time every day checking things over and over and over again.	1	2	3
11. I often have trouble finishing things because I need to make absolutely sure that everything is exactly right.	1	2	3
12. I spend far too much time arranging my things in order.	1	2	3
13. I need someone to tell me things are alright over and over again.	1	2	3
14. I find it very, very upsetting to touch garbage or garbage bins.	1	2	3
15. I check and check over and over again that my doors or windows are locked, even though I try not to do so.	1	2	3
16. I always feel I must get dressed in exactly the same order every single day.	1	2	3
17. I always count, even when doing ordinary things.	1	2	3
18. I often feel I have to ask someone the same question over and over and over again.	1	2	3
19. I am often very late because I can't finish things on time.	1	2	3

Please try to think about the three *most* upsetting **habits** that you feel you **have** to do and **can't stop**. For example, feeling that you have to wash your hands far too often, or check that your school work is just right.

1) _____

2) _____

3) _____

How much time do you spend doing these habits? Please circle the answer that best describes you.

0	1	2	3	4
None	Less than 1 hr. a day (occasionally)	1-3 hrs. a day (part of a morning or afternoon)	3-8 hrs. a day (about half the time you're awake)	More than 8 hrs. a day (almost all the time you're awake)

How much do these habits get in the way of school or doing things with friends? Please circle the answer that best describes you.

0	1	2	3	4
Not at all	A little	Somewhat	A lot	Almost always

How would you feel if prevented from carrying out your habits? How upset would you become? Please circle the answer that best describes you.

0	1	2	3	4
Not at all	A little	Somewhat	A lot	Totally

How much do you try to fight the upsetting habits? Please circle the answer that best describes you.

0	1	2	3	4
I always try to resist	I try to resist most of the time	I make some effort to resist	Even though I want to, I don't try to resist	I don't resist at all

How strong is the feeling that you have to carry out the habits? Please circle the answer that best describes you.

0	1	2	3	4
Not strong	Mild pressure to carry out habits	Strong pressure to carry out habits; hard to control	Very strong pressure to carry out habits; very hard to control	Extreme pressure to carry out habits; impossible to control

How much have you been avoiding doing anything, going any place, or being with anyone because of your upsetting habits? Please circle the answer that best describes you.

0	I	2	3	4
Not at all	A little	Somewhat	A lot	Almost always

CHOCI: Part 2

In this section, each of the questions asks you about thoughts, ideas, or pictures that keep coming into your mind even though you do not want them to do so. They may be unpleasant, silly, or embarassing. For example, some children have the repeated thought that germs or dirt are harming them or other people, or that something unpleasant may happen to them or someone special to them. These are thoughts that keep coming back, over and over again, even though you do not want them.

Please answer each question by putting a circle around the number that best describes how much you agree with the statement, or how much you think it is true of you. Please answer each item, without spending too much time on any one item. There are no right or wrong answers.

Example: I often have the same upsetting thought about death over and over again.	Not at all I	Somewhat 2	A lot 3

How much do you agree with each of the following statements?	Not at all	Somewhat	A lot
1. I often have the same upsetting thought about an accident over and over again.	I	2	3
2. I am often very upset by sudden feelings that I want to harm myself.	I	2	3
3. I often have bad thoughts that make me feel like a terrible person.	I	2	3
4. I often have horrible thoughts about my family being hurt that upset me very much.	I	2	3
5. I am often very upset by a sudden feeling that I am going to harm my family.	I	2	3
6. I often have doubts about whether I've made the right decision.	I	2	3
7. I often have the same upsetting picture in my head about death over and over again.	I	2	3
8. I often have mean thoughts that I feel are terrible, over and over again.	I	2	3
9. I often have the same horrible picture in my head about an accident.	I	2	3
10. I have upsetting sexual thoughts over and over again, even though I don't want them.	I	2	3
11. I often have horrible thoughts about going crazy.	I	2	3
12. I always think that something terrible is going to happen and it will be my fault.	I	2	3
13. I often think that my bad thoughts are as awful as actually doing the bad thing.	I	2	3

Please list the three most severe **thoughts** that you often have **and can't stop thinking about**. For example, thinking about hurting someone, or thinking bad things about God.

1) _____

2) _____

3) _____

How much time do you spend thinking about these things? Please circle the answer that best describes you.

0	I	2	3	4
None	Less than I hr. a day (occasionally)	I-3 hrs. a day (part of a morning or afternoon)	3-8 hrs. a day (about half the time you're awake)	More than 8 hrs. a day (almost all the time you're awake)

How much do these thoughts get in the way of school or doing things with friends? Please circle the answer that best describes you.

0	I	2	3	4
Not at all	A little	Somewhat	A lot	Extreme

How much do these thoughts bother or upset you? Please circle the answer that best describes you.

0	I	2	3	4
Not at all	A little	Somewhat	A lot	Extreme

How hard do you try to stop the thoughts or ignore them? Please circle the answer that best describes you.

0	I	2	3	4
I always try to resist	I try to resist most of the time	I make some effort to resist	Even though I want to, I don't try to resist	I don't resist at all

When you try to fight the thoughts, can you beat them? How much control do you have over the thoughts? Please circle the answer that best describes you.

0	I	2	3	4
Complete control	Much control	Moderate control	Little control	No control

How much have you been avoiding doing anything, going any place, or being with anyone because of your thoughts? Please circle the answer that best describes you.

0	I	2	3	4
Not at all	A little	Somewhat	A lot	Almost always

Children's Yale-Brown Obsessive Compulsive Scale (CY-BOCS)

Time 5 minutes

Ages 4–18

Time Frame Last week

Purpose Assessment of severity of obsessive and compulsive symptoms.

Commentary

The CY-BOCS is adapted from the Yale-Brown Obsessive Compulsive Scale (Y-BOCS; Goodman et al., 1989a,b) for adults. Structure, response scale, and scoring rules from the original scale were retained in the CY-BOCS, but the wording of the probing questions were changed to make them more appropriate for children. The CY-BOCS is widely used, especially in many treatment trials.

Versions

The Children's Yale-Brown Obsessive Compulsive Scale (CY-BOCS) is only available as a clinician-rated scale.

Properties

Items The CY-BOCS has five sections: instructions, obsessions checklists, severity items for obsessions, compulsions checklist, and severity items for compulsions. Both checklists are used to identify the most prominent obsessions and compulsions. The CY-BOCS comprises 10 severity items, five for obsessions and five for compulsions. The severity items assess five aspects pertaining to obsessions and compulsions: frequency, interference, distress, resistance, and control. The 10 severity items are rated on a 5-point scale with responses: none, mild, moderate, severe, and extreme for the frequency, interference, and distress items; always resists, and completely yields for the resistance items; complete control, much control, moderate control, little control, and no control for the control items.

Scales Factor analysis confirmed that the severity items can be scored on two subscales: Obsessions and Compulsions. However, factor analysis also suggested scoring on two alternative factors: Severity, which includes interference and distress items, and Disturbance, which includes frequency, resistance, and control items. In

addition, all 10 severity items can be scored on the total score.

Reliability Test–retest intraclass correlations across a 41-day interval were 0.70 and 0.76 for the Obsessions and Compulsions subscales and 0.79 for the total score in a group of children diagnosed with obsessive compulsive disorder (OCD).

Interrater intraclass correlations among four raters were 0.91 and 0.66 for the Obsessions and Compulsions subscales and 0.84 for the total score.

Cronbach's alphas were 0.87 for the total score in a first group of children diagnosed with OCD, and 0.80 and 0.82 for the Obsessions and Compulsions subscales and 0.90 for the total score in a second group.

Validity Correlations of the subscales and the total score with clinician-reported impairment, obsessions and compulsions, and with parent-reported obsessions and compulsions were high and significant.

Correlations of the CY-BOCS scales with self-reported anxiety were low and not significant and with self-reported depression, and parent-reported aggression and ADHD were moderate, but significant.

Norms No information available.

Use A copy of the CY-BOCS and further information about its use can be obtained from Wayne K. Goodman at the address below.

Key references

Goodman WK, Price LH, Rasmussen SA, et al. The Yale-Brown Obsessive Compulsive Scale, I: Development, use, and reliability. Arch Gen Psychiatry 1989; 46: 1006–11.

Goodman WK, Price LH, Rasmussen SA, et al. The Yale-Brown Obsessive Compulsive Scale, II: Validity. Arch Gen Psychiatry 1989; 46: 1012–16.

McKay D, Piacentini J, Greisberg S, et al. The Children's Yale-Brown Obsessive-Compulsive Scale: Item structure in an outpatient setting. Psychol Assess 2003; 15: 578–81.

Scahill L, Riddle MA, McSwiggin-Hardin M, et al. Children's Yale-Brown Obsessive Compulsive Scale:

Reliability and validity. J Am Acad Child Adolesc Psychiatry 1997; 36: 844–52.

Storch EA, Murphy TK, Geffken GR, et al. Factor analytic study of the Children's Yale-Brown Obsessive-Compulsive Scale. J Clin Child Adolesc Psychol 2005; 34: 312–19.

Storch EA, Murphy TK, Geffken GR, et al. Psychometric evaluation of the Children's Yale-Brown Obsessive-Compulsive Scale. Psychiatr Res 2004; 129: 91–8.

Address

Wayne K. Goodman
Department of Psychiatry
College of Medicine
University of Florida
PO Box 100256
Gainesville, FL 32610–0256
USA
wkgood@psychiatry.ufl.edu

Children's Yale-Brown Obsessive Compulsive Scale (CY-BOCS) Obsessions Checklist

Name_____   Date _____

Check all symptoms that apply. (Items marked '*' may or may not be OCD phenomena.)

Current   Past

Contamination obsessions

_____ _____ Concern with dirt, germs, certain illnesses (e.g., AIDS)
_____ _____ Concerns or disgust with bodily waste or secretions (e.g., urine, feces, saliva)
_____ _____ Excessive concern with environmental contaminants (e.g., asbestos, radiation, toxic waste)
_____ _____ Excessive concern with household items (e.g., cleaners, solvents)
_____ _____ Excessive concern about animals/insects
_____ _____ Excessively bothered by sticky substances or residues
_____ _____ Concerned will get ill because of contaminant
_____ _____ Concerned will get others ill by spreading contaminant (aggressive)
_____ _____ No concern with consequence of contamination other than how it might feel*
_____ _____ Other (describe): _____

Aggressive obsessions

_____ _____ Fear might harm self
_____ _____ Fear might harm others
_____ _____ Fear harm will come to self
_____ _____ Fear harm will come to others (may be because of something child did or did not do)
_____ _____ Violent or horrific images
_____ _____ Fear of blurting out obscenities or insults
_____ _____ Fear of doing something else embarrassing*
_____ _____ Fear will act on unwanted impulses (e.g., to stab a family member)
_____ _____ Fear will steal things
_____ _____ Fear will be responsible for something else terrible happening (e.g., fire, burglary, flood)
_____ _____ Other (describe): _____

Sexual obsessions

_____ _____ (Are you having any sexual thoughts? If yes, are they routine or are they repetitive thoughts that you would rather not have or find disturbing? If yes, are they:)
_____ _____ Forbidden or perverse sexual thoughts, images, impulses
_____ _____ Content involves homosexuality*
_____ _____ Sexual behavior towards others (aggressive)
_____ _____ Other (describe): _____

Hoarding/saving obsessions

_____ _____ Fear of losing things
_____ _____ Other (describe): _____

Magical thoughts/superstitious obsessions

_____ _____ Lucky/unlucky numbers, colors, words
_____ _____ Other (describe): _____

Somatic obsessions

_____ _____ Excessive concern with illness or disease*
_____ _____ Excessive concern with body part or aspect of appearance (e.g., dysmorphophobia)*
_____ _____ Other (describe): _____

Religious obsessions (scrupulosity)

_____ _____ Excessive concern or fear of offending religious objects (God)
_____ _____ Excessive concern with right/wrong, morality
_____ _____ Other (describe): _____

Miscellaneous obsessions

_____ _____ The need to know or remember
_____ _____ Fear of saying certain things
_____ _____ Fear of not saying just the right thing
_____ _____ Intrusive (nonviolent) images
_____ _____ Intrusive sounds, words, music, or numbers
_____ _____ Other (describe): _____

Name_____   Date _____

Check all symptoms that apply. (Items marked '*' may or may not be OCD phenomena.)

Current Past

Washing/cleaning compulsions
_____ _____   Excessive or ritualized handwashing
_____ _____   Excessive or ritualized showering, bathing, toothbrushing, grooming, toilet routine
_____ _____   Excessive cleaning of items; such as personal clothes or important objects
_____ _____   Other measures to prevent or remove contact with contaminants
_____ _____   Other (describe): _____

Checking compulsions
_____ _____   Checking locks, toys, school book/items, etc.
_____ _____   Checking associated with getting washed, dressed, or undressed
_____ _____   Checking that did not/will not harm others
_____ _____   Checking that did not/will not harm self
_____ _____   Checking that nothing terrible did/will happen
_____ _____   Checking that did not make mistake
_____ _____   Checking tied to somatic obsessions
_____ _____   Other (describe): _____

Repeating rituals
_____ _____   Rereading, erasing, or rewriting
_____ _____   Need to repeat routine activities (e.g., in/out of doorway, up/down from chair)
_____ _____   Other (describe): _____

Counting compulsions
_____ _____   Objects, certain numbers, words, etc.
_____ _____   Other (describe): _____

Ordering/arranging
_____ _____   Need for symmetry/evening up (e.g., lining items up a certain way or arranging personal items in specific patterns)
_____ _____   Other (describe): _____

Hoarding/saving compulsions
(distinguish from hobbies and concern with objects of monetary or sentimental value)
_____ _____   Difficulty throwing things away, saving bits of paper, string, etc.
_____ _____   Other (describe): _____

Excessive games/superstitious behaviors
(distinguish from age-appropriate magical games) (e.g. array of behavior, such as stepping over certain spots on a floor, touching an object/self certain number of times as a routine game to avoid something bad from happening.)
_____ _____   Other (describe): _____

Rituals involving other persons
_____ _____   The need to involve another person (usually a parent) in ritual (e.g., asking a parent to repeatedly answer the same question, making mother perform certain meal-time rituals involving specific utensils).*
_____ _____   Other (describe): _____

Miscellaneous compulsions
_____ _____   Mental rituals (other than checking/counting)
_____ _____   Need to tell, ask, or confess
_____ _____   Measures (not checking) to prevent harm to self ___; harm to others ___; terrible consequences ___
_____ _____   Ritualized eating behaviors*
_____ _____   Excessive list making*
_____ _____   Need to touch, tap, rub*
_____ _____   Need to do things (e.g., touch or arrange) until it *feels* just right)*
_____ _____   Rituals involving blinking or staring*
_____ _____   Trichotillomania (hair-pulling)*
_____ _____   Other self-damaging or self-mutilating behaviors*
_____ _____   Other (describe): _____

Children's Yale-Brown Obsessive Compulsive Scale (CY-BOCS)

CY-BOCS total (add items 1–10) _____

Patient name _____   Date _____

Patient ID _____   Rater _____

		None	Mild	Moderate	Severe	Extreme
1.	Time spent on obsessions	0	1	2	3	4

		No symptoms	Long	Moderately long	Short	Extremely short
1b.	Obsession-free interval (do not add to subtotal or total score)	0	1	2	3	4

2.	Interference from obsessions	0	1	2	3	4
3.	Distress of obsessions	0	1	2	3	4

		Always resists				Completely yields
4.	Resistance	0	1	2	3	4

		Complete control	Much control	Moderate control	Little control	No control
5.	Control over obsessions	0	1	2	3	4

Obsession subtotal (add items 1–5) _____

		None	Mild	Moderate	Severe	Extreme
6.	Time spent on compulsions	0	1	2	3	4

		No symptoms	Long	Moderately long	Short	Extremely short
6b.	Compulsion-free interval (do not add to subtotal or total score)	0	1	2	3	4

7.	Interference from compulsions	0	1	2	3	4
8.	Distress from compulsions	0	1	2	3	4

		Always resists				Completely yields
9.	Resistance	0	1	2	3	4

		Complete control	Much control	Moderate control	Little control	No control
10.	Control over compulsions	0	1	2	3	4

Compulsion subtotal (add items 6–10) _____

		Excellent				Absent
11.	Insight into O–C symptoms	0	1	2	3	4

		None	Mild	Moderate	Severe	Extreme
12.	Avoidance	0	1	2	3	4
13.	Indecisiveness	0	1	2	3	4
14.	Pathologic responsibility	0	1	2	3	4
15.	Slowness	0	1	2	3	4
16.	Pathologic doubting	0	1	2	3	4

17.	Global severity	0	1	2	3	4	5	6
18.	Global improvement	0	1	2	3	4	5	6

19.	Reliability	Excellent = 0	Good = 1	Fair = 2	Poor = 3

© Wayne K. Goodman. Reproduced by permission. Anyone who is interested in using the CY-BOCS for research or clinical practice should contact Wayne K. Goodman who can provide instructions and copies of the scale.

Leyton Obsessional Inventory – Child Version (LOI-CV)

Time 10 minutes

Ages 13–18

Time Frame Not Specified.

Purpose Assessment of obsessive and compulsive symptoms.

Commentary

The LOI-CV is an adaptation of the 69-item Leyton Obsessive Inventory for adults by Cooper (1970). The child version was shortened to reduce time needed for children to complete the scale and several items were replaced by items more appropriate for children. The card-sorting task version can also be used to observe children's obsessions and compulsions while conducting the task, but the survey form is more feasible for use in epidemiological studies.

Versions

The Leyton Obsessional Inventory-Child Version (LOI-CV) is available in three versions: A 44-item card-sorting task version, a 20-item self-report survey form which is described here, and a 11-item short version of the survey form.

Properties

Items   The LOI-CV survey form comprises 20 items that are rated on a 2-point scale with responses: yes, and no. If an item is rated yes, then this item is also rated on a 4-point interference scale with responses: this habit does not stop me from doing other things I want to do, this stops me a little or wastes a little of my time, this stops me from doing other things or wastes some of my time, and this stops me from doing a lot of things and wastes a lot of my time.

Scales   Factor analysis was used to determine the structure of the LOI-CV. Four factors were retained which are labeled: general obsessive, dirt-contamination, numbers-luck, and school. In addition, a total score is the sum of ratings of all items. Both yes ratings and interference ratings are used to compute subscale scores and the total score.

Reliability   Cronbach's alphas were 0.81 for the total score, 0.81 for general obsessive, 0.65 for both dirt-contamination and numbers-luck, and 0.49 for school in a sample of 4551 school children.

Validity   A cut-off score for interference ratings discriminated between children with an obsessive compulsive disorder and children with no diagnosis with a sensitivity of 75% and a specificity of 84%. For yes ratings, the sensitivity was 88% and the specificity 77%.

Norms   A table with items means for a total group of 4551 school children and separately for boys and girls is given in Berg et al. (1988). Cut-off scores that discriminate children with an obsessive compulsive disorder and children with no diagnosis are reported in Flament et al. (1988).

Use   The card-sorting task version of the LOI-CV can be found in Berg et al. (1986), the 20-item version in Berg et al. (1988), and the 11-item short form in Bamber et al. (2002).

Key references

Bamber D, Tamplin A, Park RJ, Kyte ZA, Goodyer IM. Development of a short Leyton Obsessional Inventory for children and adolescents. J Am Acad Child Adolesc Psychiatry 2002; 41: 1246–52.

Berg CJ, Rapoport JL, Flament M. The Leyton Obsessional Inventory-Child Version. J Am Acad Child Adolesc Psychiatry 1986; 25: 84–91.

Berg CZ, Whitaker A, Davies M, Flament MF, Rapoport JL. The survey form of the Leyton Obsessional Inventory-Child Version: Norms from an epidemiological sample. J Am Acad Child Adolesc Psychiatry 1988; 27: 759–763.

Cooper J. The Leyton Obsessional Inventory. Psychol Med 1970; 1: 48–64.

Flament MF, Whitaker A, Rapoport JL, et al. Obsessive compulsive disorder in adolescence: An epidemiological study. J Am Acad Child Adolesc Psychiatry 1988; 27: 764–71.

Leyton Obsessional Inventory – Child Version (LOI-CV) – survey form

1. Do you often feel like you have to do certain things even though you know you don't really have to?
2. Do thoughts or words ever keep going over and over in your mind?
3. Do you have to check things several times?
4. Do you hate dirt and dirty things?
5. Do you ever feel that if something has been used or touched by someone else it is spoiled for you?
6. Do you ever worry about being clean enough?
7. Are you fussy about keeping your hands clean?
8. When you put things away at night, do they have to be put away just right?
9. Do you get angry if other students mess up your desk?
10. Do you spend a lot of extra time checking your homework to make sure that it is just right?
11. Do you ever have to do things over and over a certain number of times before they seem quite right?
12. Do you ever have to count several times or go through numbers in your mind?
13. Do you ever have trouble finishing your school work or chores because you have to do something over and over again?
14. Do you have a favorite or special number that you like to count up to or do things just that number of times?
15. Do you often have a bad conscience because you've done something even though no one else thinks it is bad?
16. Do you worry a lot if you've done something not exactly the way you like?
17. Do you have trouble making up your mind?
18. Do you go over things a lot that you have done because you aren't sure that they were the right things to do?
19. Do you move or talk in just a special way to avoid bad luck?
20. Do you have special numbers or words you say, because it keeps bad luck away or bad things away?

If yes:

0–This habit does not stop me from doing other things I want to do

1–This stops me a little or wastes a little of my time

2–This stops me from doing other things or wastes some of my time

3–This stops me from doing a lot of things and wastes a lot of my time

3.3 Depression

Children's Depression Inventory (CDI)

Time CDI: 15 minutes; CDI:S: 10 minutes; CDI:P: 10 minutes; CDI:T: 10 minutes

Ages 7–17

Time Frame Last 2 weeks

Purpose Assessment of depressive problems.

Commentary

The development of the CDI started in 1977 with the Beck Depression Inventory (BDI; Beck, 1967) as starting point. Most of the BDI items were retained for the CDI and a few items pertaining to school and peer functioning were added. The CDI:S was developed using the normative data for the CDI. The CDI:P and CDI:T were developed more recently. Items of the CDI:P and CDI:T correspond to items of the CDI, but were rephrased for administration to parents and teachers.

Versions

The Children's Depression Inventory (CDI) comprises the original 27-item self-report (CDI), a 10-item short version of the self-report (CDI:S), a 17-item parent report (CDI:P), and a 12-item teacher report (CDI:T).

Properties

Items   The items of the 27-item CDI and the 10-item CDI:S are rated on 3-point scale. Each of the 3 responses of each item is labeled with a statement about a child's depressive feelings. The 17-item CDI:P and the 12-item CDI:T are rated on a 4-point scale with responses: not at all, some of the time, often, and much or most of the time.

Scales   The items of the CDI are scored on five subscales which are supported by factor analysis. The five subscales are: Negative Mood, Interpersonal Problems, Ineffectiveness, Anhedonia, and Negative Self-Esteem. In addition to the subscale scores a Total score can be calculated. The CDI:S is only scored on a Total score. The items of the CDI:P and CDI:T are scored on two subscales which are supported by factor analysis, and a Total score. The two subscales are: Emotional Problems, and Functional Problems.

Reliability   Test-retest correlations ranged from 0.66 to 0.83 across 2- to 4-week intervals, and ranged from 0.54 to 0.56 across 4- to 6-month intervals.

Cronbach's alphas ranged from 0.59 to 0.68 for the subscales of the CDI and the alpha was 0.86 for the Total score in the normative sample. Cronbach's alphas ranged from 0.59 to 0.66 for the subscales in a sample of Canadian school children. Cronbach's alpha for the CDI:S was 0.80 in the normative sample. Cronbach's alphas ranged from 0.76 to 0.86 for the subscales of the CDI:P and CDI:T and ranged from 0.86 to 0.89 for the Total scores in the normative samples and clinical samples.

Validity   The Total score of the CDI has a sensitivity of 80% and a specificity of 84% in distinguishing children with depression from children without depression. Subscale and Total scores on the CDI, CDI:P, and CDI:T were significantly higher in clinical groups than in non-clinical groups. The CDI was sensitive to change in clinical trials.

Norms   The CDI and CDI:S were standardized on ratings of 1266 school children in grades 2 through 8 from the United States. The CDI:P was standardized on 1187 ratings and the CDI:T was standardized on 631 ratings of children aged 7–17 years from the United States, Canada, and Australia. Raw scores for subscales and Total scores of the CDI, CDI:S, CDI:P, and CDI:T were converted to percentile equivalents.

Use   Rating scales enabling direct scoring, a manual, a computer program for data entry and scoring are available from the publisher at the address below. The manual contains an extensive annotated bibliography of key research studies up to 2003.

Key references

Beck AT. Depression: Clinical, experimental, and theoretical aspects. New York: Harper & Row, 1967.

Kovacs M. The Children's Depression Inventory. Psychopharmacol Bull 1985; 21:995–8.

Kovacs M. CDI Children's Depression Inventory. Technical Manual Update. North Tonawanda, NY: Multi-Health Systems Inc, 2003.

Address

Multi-Health Systems Inc.
P.O. Box 950
North Tonawanda, NY 14120-0950
USA
www.mhs.com

Children's Depression Inventory (CDI) – sample items

Item 7
☐ I hate myself.
☐ I do not like myself.
☐ I like myself.
Item 13
☐ I cannot make up my mind about things.
☐ It is hard to make up my mind about things.
☐ I make up my mind about things easily.
Item 25
☐ Nobody really loves me.
☐ I am not sure if anybody loves me.
☐ I am sure that somebody loves me.

Children's Depression Rating Scale – Revised (CDRS-R)

Time 10 minutes

Ages 6–12

Time Frame Not specified

Purpose Assessment of depressive symptoms.

Commentary

The development of the CDRS-R started in the 1970s and is modeled on the adult Hamilton Rating Scale for Depression. The CDRS-R is used as a screening instrument for assessing children's depressive symptoms and recognizing treatment needs.

Versions

The Children's Depression Rating Scale – Revised (CDRS-R) is a rating scale to be completed by clinicians.

Properties

Items   The CDRS-R comprises 17 items of which 14 are rated on a 7-point scale and 3 on a 5-point scale. All responses are numbered from 1 to 7 or from 1 to 5, but not every response has a label attached to its number. Furthermore, each item has labels for the responses that are different across all items. In addition to the ratings, a clinician can give comments about a rated symptom below each item. See the Sample Items section for two examples.

Scales   The items of the CDRS-R are scored on only one scale. The Summary Score is the simple sum of the ratings on all 17 items.

Reliability   Test–retest correlation for the Summary Score across a 2-week interval was 0.80.

Cronbach's alpha for the Summary score was 0.85 in a group of school children.

Interrater correlation between two clinicians was 0.92.

Validity   The CDRS-R Summary Score correlated 0.87 and 0.48 with clinician-reported ratings of depression. The Summary Score was also significantly associated with a Dexamethasone Suppression Test, where high CDRS-R scores indicated cortisol nonsuppression and low CDRS-R scores indicated cortisol suppression.

In a comparison of three groups of children, the group with clinical children diagnosed with depression had the highest CDRS-R Summary Scores, which were significantly higher than scores of both clinical children diagnosed with difficulties other than depression and normal children.

Norms   The CDRS-R was standardized on the ratings of 233 school children. The Summary Score is converted to a normalized T-score.

Use   A manual and rating forms are available from the publisher at the address below. Information about scoring and interpreting the CDRS-R are printed on each copy of the rating form. The manual includes a guide for parent interviews for obtaining information that can be used to complete the CDRS-R.

Key references

Poznanski EO, Cook SC, Carroll BJ. A depression rating scale for children. Pediatrics 1979; 64:442–50.

Poznanski EO, Freeman LN, Mokros HB. Children's depression rating scale-revised. Psychopharmacol Bull 1985; 21:979–89.

Poznanski EO, Mokros HB. Children's Depression Rating Scale: Manual. Los Angeles: Western Psychological Services, 1996.

Address

Western Psychological Services
12031 Wilshire Blvd.
Los Angeles, CA 90025-1251
USA
www.wpspublish.com

Children's Depression Rating Scale – Revised (CDRS-R) – sample items

6. Excessive fatigue

No unusual complaints of 'feeling tired' during the day	1
	2
Complaints of fatigue seem somewhat excessive and are not related to boredom or increased activity levels	3
	4
Daily complaints of feeling tired	5
	6
Complains of feeling tired most of the day. May voluntarily take long naps without feeling refreshed. Degree of fatigue interferes with play activities.	7

Comment

16. Listless speech

Quality of speech seems situationally sensitive without any noteworthy deviations	1
Slowed tempo, monotone, or overly soft speech	2
Slowed tempo with many pauses were he/she appears to drift. Hesitations include sighing. Voice qualities are distinctly monotonic and unanimated, and convey a sense of distress and psychic discomfort.	3
	4
Extreme sense of psychic distress exhibited in voice or by a profound sense of hollowness or emptiness. Has difficulty conducting the interview	5

Comment

Children's Depression Scale (CDS)

Time Self-report: 20–40 minutes; Parent report: 20 minutes; Short forms: 5 minutes

Ages 7–18

Time Frame Not specified

Purpose Assessment of depressive problems.

Commentary

The first edition of the CDS appeared in 1978. The items of the CDS were based on manifestations of childhood depression observed in clinical practice. The original 66-item version was shortened to 50 items for the third edition. The CDS now includes teacher and health-practitioner forms as well.

Versions

The Children's Depression Scale (CDS) is available as a self-report and a parent report. In addition to these 50-item standard scales, two short forms are available: a 10-item scale for teachers, and a 10-item scale for health practitioners.

Properties

Items The CDS comprises 50 items that are rated on a 5-point scale with responses: very wrong, wrong, don't know/not sure, right, and very right. The items of the self-report CDS are printed on 50 colored cards. Children consider each item, one at a time, and place each item in one of five boxes on which one response option is printed. The CDS for other informants are common paper-and-pencil rating scales with the same response options.

Scales The items are scored on two subscales: Depression, and Pleasure which were supported by factor analyses, although factor structures differed among some studies.

Reliability Test–retest correlations across a 1-week interval were 0.74 for both the Depression and Pleasure subscales among normal children. Test–retest correlations across a 12-week interval were 0.70 for Depression and 0.74 for Pleasure among school children.
Cronbach's alphas for the Depression subscale ranged from 0.89 to 0.94 for self-reports and from 0.92 to 0.95

for parent reports across studies. Cronbach's alphas for the Pleasure subscale ranged from 0.82 to 0.94 for self-reports and from 0.82 to 0.84 for parent reports. Cronbach's alphas for the Depression subscale were 0.72 and 0.82 for the teacher and health practitioners reports, respectively, and for the Pleasure subscale alphas were 0.72 and 0.81, respectively.

Validity The self-reported CDS correlated 0.84 with another self-reported measure of depression, and the parent-reported CDS correlated 0.80 with another parent-reported measure of depression in a sample of school children. Correlations of the self-reported Depression subscale with comparable self-reported measures of depression ranged from 0.45 to 0.76 among clinical children, and correlations of the parent-reported Depression subscale were 0.67 and 0.76 with parent-reported depression.

Scores on both the self-reported and parent-reported CDS were significantly higher for children with depression than for clinical children without depression and non-clinical children.

Norms The CDS was standardized on ratings of children from several Australian samples, clinical and non-clinical. Raw score were converted to deciles and quartiles.

Use A manual and rating scales can be obtained from the publisher at the address below.

Key references

Lang M, Tisher M. Children's Depression Scale, 3rd edn. Camberwell, Australia: ACER Press, 2004.

Tisher M, Lang-Takac E, Lang M. The Children's Depression Scale: Review of Australian and overseas experience. Aust J Psychol 1992; 44: 27–35.

Address

ACER Press
Australian Council for Educational Research LTD
19 Prospect Hill Road
Camberwell, Victoria 3124
Australia
www.acerpress.com.au

Depression Self-Rating Scale for Children (DSRS)

Time 5 minutes

Ages 8–14

Time Frame Last week

Purpose Assessment of depressive symptoms.

Commentary

Modified versions of the DSRS can be found in the literature, such as a version with added items and a version with rephrased items for adolescents.

Versions

The Depression Self-Rating Scale for Children (DSRS) is only available as self-report form.

Properties

Items The DSRS comprises 18 items that are rated on a 3-point scale with responses: mostly, sometimes, and never.

Scales Although factor analysis supported three subscales, the items of the DSRS are mostly scored on only one scale, which is a simple sum of the ratings of all 18 items.

Reliability Test–retest correlation for the DSRS score in a group of special school children was 0.80.

The split-half reliability coefficient for the DSRS score in a group of special school children was 0.86.

Validity Among clinical children, the children diagnosed with depression had significantly higher scores on the DSRS than children diagnosed with other problems.

Norms A cut-off value of 15 was established for distinguishing depressed children from non-depressed children. The cut-off value of 15 has a sensitivity of 67% and specificity of 77%.

Use No supplemental materials available.

Key references

Birleson P. The validity of depressive disorder in childhood and the development of a self-rating scale: A research report. J Child Psychol Psychiatry 1981; 22: 73–88.

Birleson P, Hudson I, Buchanan DG, Wolff S. Clinical evaluation of a self-rating scale for depressive disorder in childhood (Depression Self-Rating Scale). J Child Psychol Psychiatry 1987; 28: 43–60.

Address

Peter Birleson
Maroondah Hospital Child & Adolescent Mental Health Service
21 Ware Crescent
Ringwood East, VIC 3135
Australia
peter.birleson@maroondah.org.au

Depression Self-Rating Scale for Children (DSRS)

Instructions:

This self-rating scale was developed for children between the ages of 8 and 14 years of age. Please explain to the child that the scale is a way of getting to know how children really feel about things. Give the scale to the child with the directions below. If children have difficulty in reading any of the items, clinicians may read out the statements in a neutral tone of voice that indicates no preference in what they wish to hear.

Please read these statements and tick the answer that best describes how you have felt <u>in the past week</u>. Answer as honestly as you can. The correct answer is to say how <u>you</u> really have felt.

		Mostly	Sometimes	Never	
1.	I look forward to things as much as I used to..	[ ]	[ ]	[ ]	___
2.	I sleep very well..	[ ]	[ ]	[ ]	___
3.	I feel like crying...	[ ]	[ ]	[ ]	___
4.	I like to go out to play.....................................	[ ]	[ ]	[ ]	___
5.	I feel like running away....................................	[ ]	[ ]	[ ]	___
6.	I get tummy aches...	[ ]	[ ]	[ ]	___
7.	I have lots of energy...	[ ]	[ ]	[ ]	___
8.	I enjoy my food...	[ ]	[ ]	[ ]	___
9.	I can stick up for myself...................................	[ ]	[ ]	[ ]	___
10.	I think life isn't worth living............................	[ ]	[ ]	[ ]	___
11.	I am good at the things I do.............................	[ ]	[ ]	[ ]	___
12.	I enjoy the things I do as much as I used to...	[ ]	[ ]	[ ]	___
13.	I like talking with my family.............................	[ ]	[ ]	[ ]	___
14.	I have bad dreams...	[ ]	[ ]	[ ]	___
15.	I feel very lonely...	[ ]	[ ]	[ ]	___
16.	I am easily cheered up......................................	[ ]	[ ]	[ ]	___
17.	I feel so sad I can hardly stand it.....................	[ ]	[ ]	[ ]	___
18.	I feel very bored..	[ ]	[ ]	[ ]	___

Thank you.

___

The scale is in the public domain.

Kutcher Adolescent Depression Scale (KADS)

Time 5 minutes

Ages 12–17

Time Frame Last week

Purpose Assessment of depressive problems.

Commentary

The KADS was specifically designed to aid identification of depressed adolescents and for monitoring symptom severity over time. Its features are: assessment of core symptoms of depression, terminology containing standard words and words more commonly used in speech, measurement of frequency of occurrence of the symptoms. The KADS comes in three versions: a short 6-item version for screening purposes, an 11-item version for clinical use, and a 16-item version for clinical research in which detailed assessment of symptomatic response to treatment is needed. As a screening tool, the 6-item version performs as well as or even better than the 11-item and 16-item versions.

Versions

The Kutcher Adolescent Depression Scale (KADS) is only available as self-report, and comes in three different lengths: 6, 11, and 16 items.

Properties

Items The KADS comprises 16 stem items that are rated on a 4-point scale with the following responses for most items: hardly ever, much of the time, most of the time, and all of the time. Two items have responses with a different wording. The KADS also contains an additional probe for an item about appetite changes on which adolescents indicate whether their appetite has increased or decreased. Furthermore, the 16-item version of the KADS contains additional prompts for 10 items which ask how strong symptoms are.

Scales The total score of the KADS is formed from the simple sum of the stem item's scores.

Reliability Cronbach's alpha averaged across 7 visits in an 8-week trial was 0.82 for the 16-item version, 0.84 for the 11-item version, and 0.80 for the 6-item version.

Validity Correlations between the KADS and clinician-rated depression ranged from 0.37 to 0.42 for the 3 versions at the first visit of an 8-week trial. Mean correlations across all 7 visits ranged from 0.50 to 0.55. Correlations between the KADS and clinician-rated functioning ranged from 0.16 to 0.20 at the first visit of an 8-week trial and mean correlations across all 7 visits ranged from 0.21 to 0.25.

The KADS was sensitive to change, especially the 6-item and 11-item versions which had significantly larger percentage change scores than clinician-rated depression and functioning in an 8-week trial.

Diagnostic accuracy, as assessed against a clinician-administered diagnostic assessment instrument, was comparable among the 6-item and 16 item versions of the KADS and another self-rated measure of depression. The 6-item version outperformed the 16-item version. A cut-off score of 6 on the 6-item version has a sensitivity of 92% and a specificity of 71%.

Norms A table listing cut-off scores for the 6-item version with accompanying sensitivities, specificities, positive predictive values, and negative predictive values is given in LeBlanc et al. (2002).

Use Copies of the various KADS versions can be obtained from Stan Kutcher at the address listed below.

Key references

Brooks SJ, Krulewicz SP, Kutcher S. The Kutcher Adolescent Depression Scale: Assessment of its evaluative properties over the course of an 8-week pediatric pharmacotherapy trial. J Child Adolesc Psychopharmacol 2003; 13: 337–49.

LeBlanc JC, Almudevar A, Brooks SJ, Kutcher S. Screening for adolescent depression: Comparison of the Kutcher Adolescent Depression Scale with the Beck Depression Inventory. J Child Adolesc Psychopharmacol 2002; 12: 113–26.

Address

Stan Kutcher
Department of Psychiatry
Dalhousie University, QE II HSC
Abbie J. Lane Building
Suite 9212
5909 Veteran's Memorial Lane
Halifax, Nova Scotia B3H 2E2, Canada
stan.kutcher@dal.ca

Kutcher Adolescent Depression Scale (KADS)

Over the last week, how have you been 'on average' or 'usually' regarding the following items:

1) low mood, sadness, feeling blah or down, depressed, just can't be bothered.
   a) hardly ever
   b) much of the time
   c) most of the time
   d) all of the time

1a) if b, c or d, how strong were those feelings?
   a) hardly noticed them
   b) mild
   c) quite strong
   d) very strong

2) irritable, losing your temper easily, feeling pissed off, loosing it.
   a) hardly ever
   b) much of the time
   c) most of the time
   d) all of the time

2a) if b, c or d, how strong were those feelings?
   a) hardly noticed them
   b) mild
   c) quite strong
   d) very strong

3) Sleep difficulties > different from your usual (over the years before you got sick).

3a) trouble falling asleep, lying awake in bed.
   a) hardly ever
   b) much of the time
   c) most of the time
   d) all of the time

3b) sleeping poorly during the night, waking up, getting out of bed.
   a) hardly ever
   b) much of the time
   c) most of the time
   d) all of the time

3c) waking up too early in the morning, at least 1 hour before you want to or need to get up.
   a) hardly ever
   b) much of the time
   c) most of the time
   d) all of the time

3d) sleep during the day, taking naps, lying down to rest.
   a) hardly ever
   b) much of the time
   c) most of the time
   d) all of the time

4) feeling decreased interest in: hanging out with friends; being with your best friend; being with your spouse/boyfriend/girlfriend; going out of the house; doing school work or work; doing hobbies or sports or recreation.
   a) hardly ever
   b) much of the time
   c) most of the time
   d) all of the time

4a) if b, c or d, how strong were those feelings?
   a) hardly noticed them
   b) mild
   c) quite strong
   d) very strong

5) feelings of worthlessness, hopelessness, letting people down, not being a good person.
   a) hardly ever
   b) much of the time
   c) most of the time
   d) all of the time

5a) if b, c or d, how strong were those feelings?
   a) hardly noticed them
   b) mild
   c) quite strong
   d) very strong

6) feeling tired, feeling fatigued, low in energy, hard to get motivated, have to push to get things done, want to rest or lie down a lot.
   a) hardly ever
   b) much of the time
   c) most of the time
   d) all of the time

6a) if b, c or d, how strong were those feelings?
   a) hardly noticed them
   b) mild
   c) quite strong
   d) very strong

7) trouble concentrating, can't keep your mind on schoolwork or work, daydreaming when you should be working, hard to focus when reading, getting 'bored' with work or school.
   a) hardly ever
   b) much of the time
   c) most of the time
   d) all of the time

7a) if b, c or d, how strong was this?
   a) hardly noticed them
   b) mild
   c) quite strong
   d) very strong

8) appetite changing from usual (before you got sick); not feeling hungry, not wanting to eat or feeling really hungry, wanting to eat a lot.
   a) hardly ever
   b) much of the time
   c) most of the time
   d) all of the time
   note: increased ____ or decreased ____

8a) if b, c or d, how strong were those feelings?
   a) hardly noticed them
   b) mild
   c) quite strong
   d) very strong

9) feeling that life is not very much fun, not feeling good when usually (before getting sick) would feel good, not getting as much pleasure from fun things as usual (before getting sick).
   a) hardly ever
   b) much of the time
   c) most of the time
   d) all of the time

9a) if b, c or d, how strong are these?
   a) hardly noticed them
   b) mild
   c) quite strong
   d) very strong

10) feeling worried, nervous, panicky, tense, keyed up, anxious.
   a) hardly ever
   b) much of the time
   c) most of the time
   d) all of the time

10a) if b, c or d, how strong are these?
   a) hardly noticed them
   b) mild
   c) quite strong
   d) very strong

11) physical feelings of worry like: headaches, butterflies, nausea, tingling, restlessness, diarrhea, shakes or tremors.
   a) hardly ever
   b) much of the time
   c) most of the time
   d) all of the time

11a) if b, c or d, how strong are these?
   a) hardly noticed them
   b) mild
   c) quite strong
   d) very strong

12) interest in sex, thoughts about sex, sexual arousal (compared to before you were ill), sexual fantasies.
   a) as usual or think about it more
   b) occasionally think about it
   c) seldom think about it
   d) never think about it

13) Thoughts, plans or actions about suicide or self-harm.
   a) no thoughts or plans or actions
   b) occasional thoughts, no plans or actions
   c) frequent thoughts, no plans or actions
   d) plans and/or actions that have hurt

Mood and Feelings Questionnaire (MFQ)

Time Standard version: 10 minutes; Short version: 3 minutes

Ages 8–18

Time Frame Last two weeks

Purpose Assessment of depressive problems.

Commentary

The MFQ was developed to select children and adolescents for an epidemiological study of depression. It was designed to cover symptoms specified by DSM-III-R, but included other symptoms of clinical significance as well.

Versions

The Mood and Feelings Questionnaire (MFQ) is available as a self-report and a parent report. Both are also available as short forms (SMFQ).

Properties

Items The MFQ comprises 32 items and the SMFQ 13 items that are rated on a 3-point scale with responses: not true, sometimes true, and not true.

Scales The items of the MFQ and SMFQ are scored on a total score which is the simple sum of all item ratings.

Reliability Test–retest correlation across a 1-week interval was 0.72 for the MFQ in a sample of clinical children. Test–retest correlations of the self-report MFQ were 0.84 across a 3-week interval and 0.80 across a 3-month interval in a sample of school children.

Cronbach's alphas were 0.90 for both the parent and self-report MFQ, and 0.87 and 0.85, respectively for the SMFQ in a sample of psychiatric and pediatric patients.

Validity Correlations of the parent and self-report MFQ and SMFQ with self-reported and parent-reported depression ranged from 0.19 to 0.67. The correlations among self-reports were highest and ranged from 0.58 to 0.67.

Both the parent and self-report SMFQ significantly discriminated between pediatric and psychiatric patients. The MFQ distinguished depressed patients from non-depressed patients with a sensitivity of 88% and a specificity of 70%. The combination of parent and self-report SMFQ had a sensitivity of 70% and a specificity of 85% in distinguishing children with a depressive disorder from children without a depressive disorder.

Norms A table with means and standard deviations divided by sex of 2443 self-ratings of Norwegian school children aged 13 and 14 years is printed in Sund et al (2001).

Use The rating scales can be downloaded from the website at the address below.

Key references

Costello EJ, Angold A. Scales to assess child and adolescent depression: Checklists, screens, and nets. J Am Acad Child Adolesc Psychiatry 1988; 27: 726–37.

Messer SC, Angold A, Costello EJ, et al. Development of a short questionnaire for use in epidemiological studies of depression in children and adolescents: Factor composition and structure across development. Int J Meth Psychiatry Res 1995; 5: 251–62.

Angold A, Costello EJ, Messer SC, et al. Development of a short questionnaire for use in epidemiological studies of depression in children and adolescents. Int J Meth Psychiatry Res 1995; 5: 237–49.

Sund AM, Larsson B, Wichstrøm L. Depressive symptoms among young Norwegian adolescents as measured by the Mood and Feeling Questionnaire (MFQ). Eur Child Adolesc Psychiatry 2001; 10: 222–9.

Address

Adrian Angold
Developmental Epidemiological Program
Duke University Medical Center
Box 3454
Durham, North Carolina 27710
USA
adrian.angold@duke.edu
devepi.mc.duke.edu/MFQ.html

Reynolds Child Depression Scale (RCDS) and Reynolds Adolescent Depression Scale-2nd Edition (RADS-2)

Time RCDS: 10 minutes; RADS-2: 5 minutes

Ages RCDS: 8–12; RADS-2: 11–20

Time Frame RCDS: Last 2 weeks; RADS-2: Not specified

Purpose Assessment of depressive problems.

Commentary

The development of the RCDS and the RADS, the initial version of the RADS-2 began in 1981. The revision of the RADS was published in 2002 as the RADS-2. All items were retained in the revision, but it was standardized on a new sample. Most items on the RCDS and RADS-2 are similar, only a few are totally different, and only a few have minor differences, for example, the word kids on the RCDS was changed into students on the RADS-2.

Versions

The Reynolds Child Depression Scale (RCDS) and Reynolds Adolescent Depression Scale-2nd Edition (RADS-2) are both only available as a self-report.

Properties

Items Both the RCDS and RADS-2 comprise 30 items that are rated on a 4-point scale, except for item 30 of the RCDS which is rated on a 5-point scale that has five faces as response options. For the RCDS the responses are: almost never, sometimes, a lot of the time, and all the time. For the RADS-2 the responses are: almost never, hardly ever, sometimes, most of the time.

Scales The items of the RCDS are only scored on a total score. The items of the RADS-2 are scored on 4 subscales which were supported by factor analysis. These 4 subscales are: Dysphoric Mood, Anhedonia/Negative Affect, Negative Self-Evaluation, and Somatic Complaints. In addition to the subscales, the Depression Total is computed by summing all items.

Reliability Test–retest correlations were 0.82 across a 2-week interval and 0.85 across a 4-week interval for the total score of the RCDS in samples of school children.

Test–retest correlations across a 2-week interval ranged from 0.77 to 0.85 for the subscales and the correlation was 0.86 for the Depression Total of the RADS-2 in the standardization sample, and ranged from 0.81 to 0.87 for the subscales and the correlation was 0.89 for the Depression Total in a clinical sample.

Cronbach's alphas ranged from 0.85 to 0.91 for the total score of the RCDS across gender and age groups of the standardization sample.
Cronbach's alphas ranged from 0.78 to 0.92 for the subscales, and from 0.91 to 0.94 for the Depression Total of the RADS-2 across gender and age groups of the standardization sample. Cronbach's alphas ranged from 0.81 to 0.87 for the subscales and the alpha was 0.94 for the Total Depression of the RADS-2 in a clinical sample.

Validity Correlations of the total score of the RCDS with a comparable self-reported measure of depression ranged from 0.68 to 0.79, with self-reported anxiety ranged from 0.60 to 0.67, and with self-reported self-esteem ranged from –0.46 to –0.71. Correlations with academic abilities ranged from 0.03 to 0.16 in absolute values.

The RCDS distinguished between depressed and non-depressed children based on clinician's ratings with a sensitivity of 73% and a specificity of 97%. In a clinical trial comparing two behavioural treatments to a waiting-list control group, RCDS scores declined in both treatment groups, but not in the control group.

Correlations with self-reported depression ranged from 0.42 to 0.76 for the subscales and total scale of RADS-2. Correlations with depression scores obtained with clinical interviews with adolescents ranged from 0.47 to 0.82. Correlations with self-reported suicidal ideations and behaviors ranged from 0.39 to 0.71, with self-reported anxiety from 0.46 to 0.77, except 1 correlation of 0.22, with self-reported hopelessness from 0.48 to 0.60, and with self-reported self-esteem from 0.55 to 0.71.

Correlations of the RADS-2 with social desirability ranged from –0.19 to –0.38, and with academic achievement ranged from –0.12 to –0.22.

Adolescents diagnosed with major depressive disorder had significantly higher scores on the subscales and total score of the RADS-2 than normal adolescents matched on gender and age. The RADS-2 distinguished between these two groups with a sensitivity of 92% and a specificity of 84%.

Norms The RCDS was standardized on a school-based sample of children from grades 2–7 in the USA. Raw scores were converted to percentile ranks. The RADS-2 was standardized on a school-based sample of 3300 adolescents aged 11–20 years in the USA and Canada. Raw scores were converted to T-scores and percentile ranks.

Use A manual and rating scales for the RCDS, and a manual, rating scales, and profile sheets for the RADS-2 are available from the publisher at the address below.

Key references

Reynolds WM. RCDS Reynolds Child Depression Scale. Professional Manual. Lutz, Fl: Psychological Assessment Resources, Inc, 1989.

Reynolds WM. RADS-2 Reynolds Adolescent Depression Scale-2nd Edition. Professional Manual. Lutz, Fl: Psychological Assessment Resources, Inc, 2002.

Address

Psychological Assessment Resources, Inc.
16204 N. Florida Avenue
Lutz, FL 33549
USA
www.parinc.com

Reynolds Adolescent Depression Scale – 2nd Edition (RADS-2) – sample items

	Almost never	Hardly ever	Sometimes	Most of the time
9. I feel that no one cares about me	0	1	2	3
26. I feel worried	0	1	2	3

3.4 Suicide

Child-Adolescent Suicidal Potential Index (CASPI)

Time 10 minutes

Ages 6–18

Time Frame Last 6 months

Purpose Assessment of risks for suicidal behavior.

Commentary

The CASPI was designed to assess multiple aspects of suicicidal behavior that had been identified in empirical studies of children and adolescents.

Versions

The Child-Adolescent Suicidal Potential Index (CASPI) is available as a self-report form only.

Properties

Items   The CASPI comprises 30 items that are rated on a 2-point scale with responses: yes and no.

Scales   Factor analysis supported three subscales which are labeled: Anxious-Impulsive Depression, Suicidal Ideation or Acts, and Family Distress. In addition, the total score is the simple sum of all the items.

Reliability   Test retest correlations across a 2-week interval were 0.76 for the total score and 0.76, 0.59, 0.71 for the three subscales.
Cronbach's alphas were 0.90 for the total score and 0.86, 0.85, and 0.77 for the three subscales.

Validity   The total score and subscales correlated significantly with self-reported depression, anxiety, and hopelessness.

Mean scores for the total score and subscale scores were significantly different among three groups of children and adolescents with reported suicide attempts, reported suicide ideation, and reported no history of suicide attempts or ideation. The group of children and adolescents with suicide attempts had the highest scores on the CASPI. Children and adolescents with suicide attempts or ideation had both higher scores than children without suicidal behavior. Children and adolescents with assaultive acts or ideation had significantly higher total scores and subscale scores on the CASPI than children and adolescents without assaultive behavior.

Norms   A table with various cutoff values discriminating among children and adolescents with suicide attempts, ideation, and without suicidal behavior are reported in Pfeffer at al. (2000), together with corresponding sensitivities and specificities

Use   Copies of the scale can be obtained from Cynthia R. Pfeffer at the address below.

Key references

Pfeffer CR, Jiang H, Kakuma T. Child-Adolescent Suicidal Potential Index (CASPI): A screen for risk for early onset suicidal behavior. Psychol Assess 2000; 12: 304–18.

Address

Cynthia R. Pfeffer
New York-Presbyterian Hospital-Westchester Division
21 Bloomingdale Road
White Plains, New York 10605
USA
pfeffer2@rsl.med.cornell.edu

Multi-Attitude Suicide Tendency Scale (MAST)

Time 10 minutes

Ages 14–24

Time Frame Not specified

Purpose Assessment of suicidal behavior.

Commentary

The MAST was developed as a comprehensive, multi-facet suicidal tendency scale on the basis of a model of suicidal behavior by Orbach (see Orbach et al, 1991). The model states that suicidal behavior evolves around a basic conflict among attitudes toward life and death. There are four types of conflicting attitudes involving repulsion by and attraction toward life as well as repulsion and attraction toward death. The balance between these attitudes is a determining factor in the move to suicide (Orbach et al., 1991).

Versions

The Multi-Attitude Suicide Tendency Scale (MAST) is only available as a self-report.

Properties

Items   The MAST comprises 30 items that are rated on a 5-point scale with responses: strongly disagree, disagree, neither agree or disagree, agree, strongly agree.

Scales   Factor analysis was used to determine the dimensions of the MAST. The items can be scored on four subscales which are labeled: Attraction to Life (AL), Repulsion by Life (RL), Attraction to Death (AD), and Repulsion by Death (RD).

Reliability   Cronbach's alphas ranged from 0.76 to 0.83 for the 4 subscales in a combination of suicidal, psychiatric, and normative groups.

Validity   Correlations between the 4 subscales and self-reported suicide potential were –0.66, 0.64, 0.48, and

0.28 for AL, RL, AD, and RD, respectively. Only the correlation that involved RD was not significant.

Comparisons among suicidal, psychiatric, and normative groups revealed significantly higher scores for the normative group for AL, higher scores for the suicidal group for RL and AD than the other groups. Only RD was not significantly different among the 3 groups. Comparisons between attempters and ideators revealed higher scores of AL for ideators and higher scores of RL for attempters.

Norms   A table with means and standard deviations of the 4 subscale scores for a normative group of 90 Israeli adolescents can be found in Orbach et al. (1991), and a similar table for American adolescents in Osman et al. (1994).

Use   The MAST can be obtained from Israel Orbach at the address below.

Key references

Orbach I, Milstein I, Har-Even D, et al. A Multi-Attitude Suicide Tendency Scale for adolescents. Psychol Assess 1991; 3: 398–404.

Osman A, Barrios FX, Grittmann LR, Osman JR. The Multi-Attitude Suicide Tendency Scale: Psychometric characteristics in an American sample. J Clin Psychol 1993; 49: 701–8.

Osman A, Barrios FX, Panak WF, Osman JR. Validation of the Multi-Attitude Suicide Tendency Scale in an adolescent sample. J Clin Psychol 1994; 50: 847–55.

Address

Israel Orbach
Department of Psychology
Bar-Ilan University
Ramat-Gan 52900
Israel
orbachi@mail.biu.ac.il

Mult-Attitude Suicide Tendency Scale (MAST)

The following are statements about life and death. Will you be so kind as to respond to them. There are no right or wrong answers. We are interested in your **personal** opinion if you agree or disagree with each statement.

Please read each statement and check the number which represents your personal opinion in the following way:

1. when you strongly disagree
2. when you disagree
3. when you neither agree or disagree
4. when you agree
5. when you strongly agree

	Description	strongly disagree	disagree	neither agree or disagree	agree	strongly agree
1.	Most of the time I feel happy	1	2	3	4	5
2.	Life seem to be one long and difficult struggle	1	2	3	4	5
3.	I fear the idea that there is no return from death	1	2	3	4	5
4.	I fear death because all my mental and spiritual activity will stop	1	2	3	4	5
5.	Even though things may be tough at times, I think it's worth living	1	2	3	4	5
6.	I feel that close people make me feel good	1	2	3	4	5
7.	I fear death because my identity will disappear	1	2	3	4	5
8.	I know people who died and I believe that I will meet them when I die	1	2	3	4	5
9.	I don't ask for help even when things are very tough for me	1	2	3	4	5
10.	Thinking about death gives me the shivers	1	2	3	4	5
11.	I am afraid of death because my body will rot	1	2	3	4	5
12.	I fear death because it means that I will not be able to experience and think anymore	1	2	3	4	5
13.	I can see myself as being very successful in the future	1	2	3	4	5
14.	I feel that I am not important to my family	1	2	3	4	5
15.	Sometimes I feel that my family will be better off without me	1	2	3	4	5
16.	Sometimes I feel that my problems can't be solved	1	2	3	4	5
17.	Death can change things for the better	1	2	3	4	5
18.	I like to do many things	1	2	3	4	5
19.	Death is actually eternal life	1	2	3	4	5
20.	The thought that one day I will die frightens me	1	2	3	4	5
21.	I don't like to spend time with my family	1	2	3	4	5
22.	Many problems can be solved by death only	1	2	3	4	5
23.	I believe that death can bring a great relief for suffering	1	2	3	4	5
24.	I fear death because all my plans will come to an end	1	2	3	4	5
25.	I am very hopeful	1	2	3	4	5
26.	In some situations it is better to die than go on living	1	2	3	4	5
27.	Death can be a state of rest and calm	1	2	3	4	5
28.	I enjoy many things in life	1	2	3	4	5
29.	Death frightens me more than anything else	1	2	3	4	5
30.	No one really loves me	1	2	3	4	5

Positive and Negative Suicide Ideation Inventory (PANSI)

Time 5 minutes

Ages 14–19

Time Frame Last 2 weeks

Purpose Assessment of positive and negative thoughts related to suicide.

Commentary

While most suicide scales only assess negative thoughts related to suicide, the PANSI was developed to assess both positive and negative thoughts. The development of the PANSI was motivated by the clinical assumption that many negative thoughts associated with few positive thoughts form significant risk factors for suicidal behavior.

Versions

The Positive and Negative Suicide Ideation Inventory (PANSI) is only available as a self-report.

Properties

Items   The PANSI comprises 14 items that are rated on a 5-point scale with responses: none of the time, very rarely, some of the time, a good part of the time, most of the time.

Scales   Factor analysis supported two subscales which are labeled: Positive Ideation, and Negative Suicide Ideation.

Reliability   Test–retest correlations across a 2-week interval were 0.69 for Positive Ideation and 0.79 for Negative Suicide Ideation among adolescent psychiatric inpatients.

Cronbach's alphas for Positive Ideation and Negative Suicide Ideation, respectively were 0.80 and 0.94 among undergraduates, 0.81 and 0.94 among high school students, and 0.89 and 0.96 among adolescent psychiatric inpatients.

Validity   Correlations of Positive Ideation with self-reported measures of suicidal behaviors among undergraduates ranged from –0.21 to –0.47 and those of

Negative Suicide Ideation ranged from 0.39 to 0.61. Among adolescent psychiatric inpatients Positive Ideation correlated –0.34 with self-reported suicidal behavior and 0.39 with a self-reported attitude toward life, while these correlations were 0.50 and –0.34, respectively for Negative Suicide Ideation.

Comparisons among three groups of adolescents with different suicide risks revealed that for Negative Suicide Ideation adolescent psychiatric inpatients with suicide risk had significantly higher scores than high school students with suicide risk. Both groups with suicide risk had significantly higher scores than high school students without suicide risk. For Positive Ideation both groups with suicide risk had significantly lower scores than high school students without suicide risk. ROC analysis was used to determine cut-off scores that could be used to distinguish groups with different suicide risks. The PANSI distinguished between the psychiatric risk group and the high school control group with a sensitivity of 73% and a specificity of 81% for Positive Ideation, and 90% and 93%, respectively for Negative Suicide Ideation. For distinguishing between the high school risk group and the high school control group sensitivity and specificity were 76% and 81%, respectively for Positive Ideation, and 90% and 80%, respectively for Negative Suicide Ideation.

Comparisons among adolescent psychiatric inpatients who were classified into suicide attempters (SA), severe at risk for suicide (SAR), and nonsuicidal (NS) revealed that the SA group had significantly higher scores for Negative Suicide Ideation and significantly lower scores for Positive Ideation than the SAR and NS groups.

Norms   Osman et al. (2003) reported a table with means and standard deviations of the subscale scores of 217 high school students separately and combined for boys and girls.

Use   The PANSI can be downloaded from the website at the address below.

Key references

Osman A, Barrios FX, Gutierrez PM, et al. The Positive and Negative Suicide Ideation (PANSI) Inventory: Psychometric evaluation with adolescent psychiatric inpatient samples. J Pers Assess 2002; 79: 512–30.

Osman A, Gutierrez PM, Jiandani J, et al. A preliminary validation of the Positive and Negative Suicide Ideation (PANSI) Inventory with normal adolescent samples. J Clin Psychol 2003; 59: 493–512.

Osman A, Gutierrez PM, Kopper BA, Barrios FX, Chiros CE. The Positive and Negative Suicide Ideation Inventory: Development and validation. Psychol Rep 1998; 82: 783–93.

Address

Agustine Osman
University of Northern Iowa
Department of Psychology
Psychology I, Room 104
Cedar Falls, IA 50614–0505
USA
augustine.osman@uni.edu
www.uni.edu/osman

3.5 Eating Disorders

Anorectic Behavior Observation Scale (ABOS)

Time 5 minutes

Ages 12–24

Time Frame Last month

Purpose Assessment of eating behaviors and attitudes.

Commentary

The ABOS was developed as a parent-report form, because parents' description of their children's eating behavior can yield more diagnostic clues than the children's reports.

Versions

The Anorectic Behavior Observation Scale (ABOS) is only available as a parent-report form, but can also be completed by spouses.

Properties

Items   The ABOS comprises 30 items that are rated on a 3-point scale with responses: yes, no, and ?.

Scales   Factor analysis supported three factors, although the original factore structure could not be replicated in a Japanese sample. The items are scored on three subscales which are labeled: Eating behavior, Bulimic-like behavior, and Hyperactivity.

Reliability   Cronbach's alphas were 0.80 for the subscale Eating behavior, 0.69 for Bulimic-like behavior, and 0.69 for Hyperactivity.

Validity   Items of the ABOS correlated significantly with corresponding items of self-report and clinician-report measures of eating behavior.

Norms   A cut-off value of 19 discriminates with a sensitivity of 90% and a specificity of 90% between women diagnosed with anorexia nervosa or bulimia nervosa and women recruited from secondary schools and college.

Use   No supplementary materials available.

Key references

Uehara T, Takeuchi K, Ohmori I, et al. Factor-analytic study of the Anorectic Behavior Observation Scale in Japa: Comparsion with the original Belgian study. Psychiatry Res 2002; 111: 41–246.

Vandereycken W. Validity and reliability of the Anorectic Behavior Observation Scale for parents. Acta Psychiatr Scand 1992; 85: 163–6.

Address

Walter Vandereycken
Department of Psychology
University of LeuvenTiensestraat 102
B-3000 Leuven
Belgium
walter.vandereycken@psy.kuleuven.ac.be

Anorectic Behavior Observation Scale (ABOS)

Name of patient: _____   Date: _____

Completed by: ○ both parents together
                 ○ mother
                 ○ father
                 ○ spouse
                 ○ someone else (who?.......................)

Instructions

Rate the following items on the basis of observations of the patient made during the last month at home. Rate an item 'Yes' or 'No' only if you are sure about it (for instance, if you yourself saw it happening). Rate '?' if you are not sure (for instance, if you did not have the opportunity to observe it for yourself, if you only heard about it or if you can only suppose that it happened).

		Yes	No	?
1.	Avoids eating with others or delays as much as possible before coming to the dinner table	( )	( )	( )
2.	Shows obvious signs of tension at mealtimes	( )	( )	( )
3.	Shows anger or hostility at mealtimes	( )	( )	( )
4.	Begins by cutting up food into small pieces	( )	( )	( )
5.	Complains that there is too much food or that it's too rich (fattening)	( )	( )	( )
6.	Exhibits unusual 'food faddism'	( )	( )	( )
7.	Attempts to bargain about food (for example, 'I'll eat this if I don't have to eat that')	( )	( )	( )
8.	Picks at food or eats very slowly	( )	( )	( )
9.	Prefers diet products (with low calorie content)	( )	( )	( )
10.	Seldom mentions being hungry	( )	( )	( )
11.	Likes to cook or help in the kitchen, but avoids tasting or eating	( )	( )	( )
12.	Vomits after meals	( )	( )	( )
13.	Conceals food in napkins, handbags or clothes during mealtimes	( )	( )	( )
14.	Disposes of food (out of window, into dustbin or down sink or toilet)	( )	( )	( )
15.	Conceals or hoards food in own room or elsewhere	( )	( )	( )
16.	Eats when alone or secretly (for example at night)	( )	( )	( )
17.	Dislikes visiting others or going to parties because of the 'obligation' to eat	( )	( )	( )
18.	Has sometimes difficulties in stopping eating or eats unusually large amounts of food or sweets	( )	( )	( )
19.	Complains a lot about constipation	( )	( )	( )
20.	Frequently takes laxatives (purgatives) or asks for them	( )	( )	( )
21.	Claims to be too fat regardless of weight loss	( )	( )	( )
22.	Often speaks about slimming, dieting or ideal body forms	( )	( )	( )
23.	Often leaves the table during mealtimes (for example, to get something in the kitchen)	( )	( )	( )
24.	Stands, walks or runs about whenever possible	( )	( )	( )
25.	Is as active as possible (for example, clearing tables or cleaning the room)	( )	( )	( )
26.	Does a lot of physical exercise or sport	( )	( )	( )
27.	Studies or works diligently	( )	( )	( )
28.	Is seldom tired and takes little or no rest	( )	( )	( )
29.	Claims to be normal, healthy or even better than ever	( )	( )	( )
30.	Is reluctant to see a doctor or refuses medical examinations	( )	( )	( )

Children's Eating Attitude Test (ChEAT)

Time 5 minutes

Ages Grade 3–8

Time Frame Not specified.

Purpose Assessment of eating behavior.

Commentary

The ChEAT is a modified version of the Eating Attitudes Test (EAT) of Garner and Garfinkle (1979).

Versions

The Children's Eating Attitude Test (ChEAT) is available as a self-report form only.

Properties

Items   The ChEAT comprises 26 items that are rated on a 6-point scale with responses: always, very often, often, sometimes, rarely, and never.

Scales   The items of the ChEAT are mostly scored on the total score only which is the simple sum of all item ratings. However, factor analysis supported three factors similar to the factors of the original EAT. The subscales derived from these factors are: dieting, restricting and purging, and food preoccupation.

Reliability   Test–retest correlation across a 3-week interval was 0.81 for the total score in elementary school children. Cronbach's alphas for the total score were 0.76 in elementary school children and 0.87 in middle school children.

Validity   The ChEAT correlated significantly with self-reported weight management behavior and self-reported body dissatisfaction.

Children who had tried to lose weight, felt too fat, and thought that their friends would like them more if they were thinner, had significantly higher total scores on the ChEAT.

Norms   The mean total score and its standard deviation for 318 elementary schoolchildren can be found in Maloney et al. (1989). A table with raw scores and converted to percentiles as well as the mean total score and its standard deviation for 308 middle school girls can be found in Smolak and Levine (1994).

Use   Copies of the ChEAT can be found in Maloney et al. (1988, 1989).

Key references

Garner DM, Garfinkle PE. The Eating Attitude Test: An index of the symptoms of anorexia nervosa. Psychol Med 1979; 9: 273–9.

Maloney MJ, McGuire, J, Daniels, SR. Reliability testing of a children's version of the Eating Attitude Test. J Am Acad Child Adolesc Psychiatry 1988; 27: 541–3.

Maloney MJ, McGuire, J, Daniels, SR, Specker B. Dieting behavior and eating attitudes in children. Pediatrics 1989; 84: 482–9.

Smolak L, Levine MP. Psychometric properties of the Children's Eating Attitude Test. Int J Eat Disord 1994; 16: 275–82.

Address

Michael J. Maloney
3002 Highland Avenue, Suite B
Cincinnati, OH 45219–2315
USA

Children's Eating Attitude Test (ChEAT)

		Always	Very often	Often	Sometimes	Rarely	Never
1.	I am scared about being overweight	(3)	(2)	(1)	(0)	(0)	(0)
2.	I stay away from eating when I am hungry	(3)	(2)	(1)	(0)	(0)	(0)
3.	I think about food a lot of the time	(3)	(2)	(1)	(0)	(0)	(0)
4.	I have gone on eating binges where I feel that I might not be able to stop	(3)	(2)	(1)	(0)	(0)	(0)
5.	I cut my food into small pieces	(3)	(2)	(1)	(0)	(0)	(0)
6.	I am aware of the energy (calorie) content in foods that I eat	(3)	(2)	(1)	(0)	(0)	(0)
7.	I try to stay away from foods such as breads, potatoes, and rice	(3)	(2)	(1)	(0)	(0)	(0)
8.	I feel that others would like me to eat more	(3)	(2)	(1)	(0)	(0)	(0)
9.	I vomit after I have eaten	(3)	(2)	(1)	(0)	(0)	(0)
10.	I feel very guilty after eating	(3)	(2)	(1)	(0)	(0)	(0)
11.	I think a lot about wanting to be thinner	(3)	(2)	(1)	(0)	(0)	(0)
12.	I think about burning up energy (calories) when I exercise	(3)	(2)	(1)	(0)	(0)	(0)
13.	Other people think I am too thin	(3)	(2)	(1)	(0)	(0)	(0)
14.	I think a lot about having fat on my body	(3)	(2)	(1)	(0)	(0)	(0)
15.	I take longer than others to eat my meals	(3)	(2)	(1)	(0)	(0)	(0)
16.	I stay away from foods with sugar in them	(3)	(2)	(1)	(0)	(0)	(0)
17.	I eat diet foods	(3)	(2)	(1)	(0)	(0)	(0)
18.	I think that food controls my life	(3)	(2)	(1)	(0)	(0)	(0)
19.	I can show self-control around food	(3)	(2)	(1)	(0)	(0)	(0)
20.	I feel that others pressure me to eat	(3)	(2)	(1)	(0)	(0)	(0)
21.	I give too much time and thought to food	(3)	(2)	(1)	(0)	(0)	(0)
22.	I feel uncomfortable after eating sweets	(3)	(2)	(1)	(0)	(0)	(0)
23.	I have been dieting	(3)	(2)	(1)	(0)	(0)	(0)
24.	I like my stomach to be empty	(3)	(2)	(1)	(0)	(0)	(0)
25.	I enjoy trying new rich foods	(3)	(2)	(1)	(0)	(0)	(0)
26.	I have the urge to vomit after eating	(3)	(2)	(1)	(0)	(0)	(0)

Children's Eating Behavior Inventory (CEBI)

Time 15 minutes

Ages 2–12

Time Frame Not specified

Purpose Assessment of eating behavior.

Commentary

The CEBI was constructed to assess eating and mealtime problems for which no instrument was available at that time. It was developed according to a framework based on a transactional and systemic understanding of parent-child relationships.

Versions

The Children's Eating Behavior Inventory (CEBI) is only available as a parent-report form.

Properties

Items   The CEBI comprises 40 items that are rated on a 5-point scale with responses: never, seldom, sometimes, often, and always. In addition, respondents are asked whether the behavior assessed in each item is a problem for them rated on a 2-point scale with responses: yes, and no.

Scales   The items of the CEBI are scored on the total eating problem score, which is the simple sum of the ratings of all items, and on the number of items to be perceived as a problem, which is the count of yes responses, but can also be expressed as a percentage.

Reliability   Test–retest correlations across a 4- to 6-week interval were 0.87 for the total eating problem score, and 0.84 for the percentage of items perceived to be a problem in a group of clinical and normal children.

Cronbach's alphas ranged from 0.58 to 0.76 in four subgroups of children.

Validity   Total eating problem scores were significantly higher for a clinical group than for a non-clinical group. The proportion of items that was perceived to be a problem was also higher for the clinical group than for the non-clinical group.

Norms   Based on the percentage of items perceived to be a problem, a cutoff value of 16% is indicative of having an eating problem.

Use   No supplementary materials available.

Key references

Archer LA, Rosenbaum PL, Streiner DL. The Children's Eating Behavior Inventory: Reliability and validity results. J Pediatr Psychol 1991; 16: 629–42.

Address

Lynda A. Archer
414-1 Young Street
Hamilton, Ontario L8N 1T8
Canada

Children's Eating Behavior Inventory (CEBI)

Child's name _____   Age _____/_____   Sex M F
                                                      Years Months

How often does this happen?

	Never	Seldom	Sometimes	Often	Always	Is this a problem for you?	
	1	2	3	4	5		
1. My child chews food as expected for his/her age	1	2	3	4	5	Yes	No
2. My child helps to set the table	1	2	3	4	5	Yes	No
3. My child watches TV at meals	1	2	3	4	5	Yes	No
4. I feed my child if he/she doesn't eat	1	2	3	4	5	Yes	No
5. My child takes more than half an hour to eat his/her meals	1	2	3	4	5	Yes	No
6. Relatives complain about my child's eating	1	2	3	4	5	Yes	No
7. My child enjoys eating	1	2	3	4	5	Yes	No
8. My child asks for food which he/she shouldn't have	1	2	3	4	5	Yes	No
9. My child feeds him/her self as expected for his/her age	1	2	3	4	5	Yes	No
10. My child gags at mealtimes	1	2	3	4	5	Yes	No
11. I feel confident my child eats enough	1	2	3	4	5	Yes	No
12. I find our meals stressful	1	2	3	4	5	Yes	No
13. My child vomits at mealtimes	1	2	3	4	5	Yes	No
14. My child takes food between meals without asking	1	2	3	4	5	Yes	No
15. My child comes to the table 1 or 2 minutes after I call	1	2	3	4	5	Yes	No
16. My child chokes at mealtimes	1	2	3	4	5	Yes	No
17. My child eats quickly	1	2	3	4	5	Yes	No
18. My child makes foods for him/her self when not allowed	1	2	3	4	5	Yes	No
19. I fet upset when my child doesn't eat	1	2	3	4	5	Yes	No
20. At home my child eats food he/she shouldn't have	1	2	3	4	5	Yes	No
21. My child eats foods that taste different	1	2	3	4	5	Yes	No
22. I let my child have snacks between meals if he/she doesn't eat at meals	1	2	3	4	5	Yes	No
23. My child uses cutlery as expected for his/her age	1	2	3	4	5	Yes	No
24. At friends' homes my child eats food he/she shouldn't eat	1	2	3	4	5	Yes	No
25. My child asks for food between meals	1	2	3	4	5	Yes	No
26. I get upset when I think about our meals	1	2	3	4	5	Yes	No
27. My child eats chunky foods	1	2	3	4	5	Yes	No
28. My child lets food sit in his/her mouth	1	2	3	4	5	Yes	No
29. At dinner I let my child choose the foods he/she wants from what is served	1	2	3	4	5	Yes	No

If you are a single parent skip to number 34

30. My child's behavior at meals upsets my spouse	1	2	3	4	5	Yes	No
31. I agree with my spouse about how much our child should eat	1	2	3	4	5	Yes	No
32. My child interrupts conversations with my spouse at meals	1	2	3	4	5	Yes	No
33. I get upset with my spouse at meals	1	2	3	4	5	Yes	No
34. My child eats when upset	1	2	3	4	5	Yes	No
35. My child says he/she is hungry	1	2	3	4	5	Yes	No
36. My child says she/he'll get fat if she/he eats too much	1	2	3	4	5	Yes	No
37. My child helps to clear the table	1	2	3	4	5	Yes	No
38. My child hides food	1	2	3	4	5	Yes	No
39. My child brings toys or books to the table	1	2	3	4	5	Yes	No

If you have only one child skip number 40

40. My child's behavior at meals upsets our other children	1	2	3	4	5	Yes	No

Please check to see that you have answered *all* the items.

Have you circled a yes or no for each item? Thank you.

Children's Eating Behaviour Questionnaire (CEBQ)

Time 10 minutes

Ages 2–11

Time Frame Not specified

Purpose Assessment of eating style.

Commentary

The CEBQ is a measure of eating style for research into the early precursors of obesity or eating disorders.

Versions

The Children's Eating Behaviour Questionnaire (CEBQ) is only available as parent-report form.

Properties

Items The CEBQ comprises 35 items that are rated on a 5-point scale with responses: never, seldom, sometimes, often, and always.

Scales Factor analysis supported 7 factors, but one factor was maintained as two subscales as these dimensions (the provisional factors satiety sensitivity and speed of eating) might usefully be separated for some purposes. Therefore, the items of the CEBQ are scored on 8 subscales, which are labeled: Food responsiveness, Enjoyment of food, Emotional overeating, Desire to drink, Satiety responsiveness, Slowness in eating, Emotional undereating, and Fussiness.

Reliability Test–retest correlations of ratings by parents of community children across a 2-week interval were 0.52 for Emotional overeating, and 0.64 for Emotional undereating, and ranged from 0.83 to 0.87 for the rest of the subscales.

Cronbach's alphas ranged from 0.72 to 0.91 in two samples of community children. Subscales Emotional overeating and Emotional undereating had Cronbach's alphas from 0.72 to 0.79 in both samples, subscales Satiety Responsiveness and Slowness in eating 0.74 in one sample, and the rest of the subscales greater than 0.80.

Validity No information available.

Norms A table with means and standard deviations divided by gender and age groups of 400 ratings by parents of community children is given in Wardle et al. (2001).

Use No supplemental materials available.

Key references

Wardle J, Guthrie CA, Sanderson, Rapoport L. Development of the Children's Eating Behaviour Questionnaire. J Child Psychol Psychiatry 2001; 42: 963–70.

Address

Jane Wardle
Cancer Research UK Health Behaviour Unit
Department of Epidemiology and Public Health
University College London
Gower Street
London WC1E 6BT
United Kingdom
j.wardle@ucl.ac.uk

Child Eating Behaviour Questionnaire (CEBQ)

Please read the following statements and tick the boxes most appropriate to your child's eating behaviour.

	Never	Rarely	Sometimes	Often	Always	
My child loves food	☐	☐	☐	☐	☐	EF
My child eats more when worried	☐	☐	☐	☐	☐	EOE
My child has a big appetite	☐	☐	☐	☐	☐	SR*
My child finishes his/her meal quickly	☐	☐	☐	☐	☐	SE*
My child is interested in food	☐	☐	☐	☐	☐	EF
My child is always asking for a drink	☐	☐	☐	☐	☐	DD
My child refuses new foods at first	☐	☐	☐	☐	☐	FF
My child eats slowly	☐	☐	☐	☐	☐	SE
My child eats less when angry	☐	☐	☐	☐	☐	EUE
My child enjoys tasting new foods	☐	☐	☐	☐	☐	FF*
My child eats less when s/he is tired	☐	☐	☐	☐	☐	EUE
My child is always asking for food	☐	☐	☐	☐	☐	FR
My child eats more when annoyed	☐	☐	☐	☐	☐	EOE
If allowed to, my child would eat too much	☐	☐	☐	☐	☐	FR
My child eats more when anxious	☐	☐	☐	☐	☐	EOE
My child enjoys a wide variety of foods	☐	☐	☐	☐	☐	FF*
My child leaves food on his/her plate at the end of a meal	☐	☐	☐	☐	☐	SR
My child takes more than 30 minutes to finish a meal	☐	☐	☐	☐	☐	SE
Given the choice, my child would eat most of the time	☐	☐	☐	☐	☐	FR
My child looks forward to mealtimes	☐	☐	☐	☐	☐	EF
My child gets full before his/her meal is finished	☐	☐	☐	☐	☐	SR
My child enjoys eating	☐	☐	☐	☐	☐	EF
My child eats more when she is happy	☐	☐	☐	☐	☐	EUE
My child is difficult to please with meals	☐	☐	☐	☐	☐	FF
My child eats less when upset	☐	☐	☐	☐	☐	EUE
My child gets full up easily	☐	☐	☐	☐	☐	SR
My child eats more when s/he has nothing else to do	☐	☐	☐	☐	☐	EOE
Even if my child is full up s/he finds room to eat his/her favourite food	☐	☐	☐	☐	☐	FR
If given the chance, my child would drink continuously throughout the day	☐	☐	☐	☐	☐	DD
My child cannot eat a meal if s/he has had a snack just before	☐	☐	☐	☐	☐	SR
If given the chance, my child would always be having a drink	☐	☐	☐	☐	☐	DD
My child is interested in tasting food s/he hasn't tasted before	☐	☐	☐	☐	☐	FF*
My child decides that s/he doesn't like a food, even without tasting it	☐	☐	☐	☐	☐	FF
If given the chance, my child would always have food in his/her mouth	☐	☐	☐	☐	☐	FR
My child eats more and more slowly during the course of a meal	☐	☐	☐	☐	☐	SE

Scoring of the CEBQ

(Never = 1, Rarely = 2, Sometimes = 3, Often = 4, Always = 5)

Food responsiveness	=	item mean FR
Emotional over-eating	=	item mean EOE
Enjoyment of food	=	item mean EF
Desire to drink	=	item mean DD
Satiety responsiveness	=	item mean SR
Slowness in eating	=	item mean SE
Emotional under-eating	=	item mean EUE
Food fussiness	=	item mean FF

*Reversed items

Questionnaire of Eating and Weight Patterns (QEWP)

Time 5 minutes

Ages 10–18

Time Frame Last 6 months.

Purpose Assessment of eating behavior.

Commentary

The QEWP-A and QEWP-P are modified versions of the Questionnaire of Eating and Weight Patterns (QEWP) of Spitzer et al (1992). The QEWP was developed to assess aspects of binge eating disorder which was introduced as a diagnostic category in the DSM-IV. The original items of the QEWP were retained while substituting difficult words with simpler synonyms for the adolescent version.

Versions

The Questionnaire of Eating and Weight Patterns (QEWP) is available as a self-report form completed by adolescents (QEWP-A) and as a parent-completed form (QEWP-P).

Properties

Items The QEWP comprises 12 stem items of which several are followed up with detail items. Most items are rated on a 2-point scale with responses yes and no. Most other items are rated on a 5-point scale. Those about how often behaviors occur have responses: less than 1 day a week, one day a week, two or three days a week, four or five days a week, and almost every day. Those about feeling bad have responses: not bad at all, just a little bad, pretty bad, very bad, and very, very bad.

Scales The ratings on the QEWP items are aggregated into three diagnostic categories: no diagnosis, nonclinical binging, and binge eating disorder.

Reliability Test–retest reliability assessed with a phi coefficient was 0.42 across a 3-week interval. The stability of diagnostic categories was higher for males than for females, who changed in 33% of the cases from the nonclinical binging to the no diagnosis category.

The kappa coefficient as a measure of agreement between self-reported and parent-reported diagnostic categories was 0.19. The concordance between adolescents and parents was 82% for the no-diagnosis category, 16% for the nonclinical binging category, and 25% for the binge eating disorder category.

Validity Children in the binge eating disorder category had significantly higher scores on self-reported depression and self-reported behaviors associated with eating disorders than children in the no diagnosis and nonclinical binging categories. In addition, the children in the nonclinical binging category had significantly higher scores on depression than the children in the no-diagnosis group.

Norms No information reported.

Use Both the QEWP-A and QEWP-P can be found in Johnson et al. (1999).

Key references

Johnson WG, Grieve FG, Adams CD, Sandy J. Measuring binge eating in adolescents: Adolescent and parent versions of the Questionnaire of Eating and Weight Patterns. Int J Eat Disord 1999; 26: 301–14.

Johnson WG, Kirk AA, Reed AE. Adolescent version of the Questionnaire of Eating and Weight Patterns: Reliability and gender differences. Int J Eat Disord 2000; 29: 94–6.

Spitzer RL, Devlin M, Walsh BT, Hassin D, Wing R, Marcus M, Stunkard A, Wadden T, Yanovski S, Agras S, Mitchell J, Nonas C. Binge eating disorder: A multi-site field trial of the diagnostic criteria. Int J Eat Disord 1992; 11: 191–203.

Address

William G. Johnson
Department of Psychiatry and Human Behavior
University of Mississippi Medical Center
2500 North State Street
Jackson, MS 39216
USA
wjohnson@psychiatry.umsmed.edu

Questionnaire of Eating and Weight Patterns (QEWP)

Adolescent version: self-report

1. During the past 6 months, did you ever eat what most people, like your friends, would think was a *really big* amount of food?
   1 YES   2 NO   (IF NO: Go to question #5)
   Did you ever eat a *really big* amount of food within a short time (2 hours or less)?
   1 YES   2 NO   (IF NO: Go to question #5)

2. When you ate a *really big* amount of food, did you ever feel that you could not stop eating? Did you feel that you could not control what or how much you were eating?
   1 YES   2 NO   (IF NO: Go to question #5)

3. During the past 6 months, how often did you eat a *really* big amount of food with the feeling that your eating was out of control?
   There may have been some weeks when you did not eat this way at all. And some weeks you may have eaten like this a lot. But, *in general*, how often did this happen?
   1 Less than 1 day a week
   2 One day a week
   3 Two or three days a week
   4 Four of five days a week
   5 Almost every day

4. When you ate a *really big* amount of food and you could not control your eating, did you:
   a) Eat *very fast*?   Yes   No
   b) Eat until your stomach hurt or you felt sick in your stomach?   Yes   No
   c) Eat really *big amounts* of food even when you were not hungry?   Yes   No
   d) Eat really *big amounts* of food during the day without regular meals like breakfast, lunch, dinner?   Yes   No
   e) Eat by yourself because you did not want anyone to see how much you ate?   Yes   No
   f) Feel *really bad* about yourself after eating a lot of food?   Yes   No

5. During the past 6 months, how bad did you feel when you ate too much or more food than you think is best for you?
   1 Not bad at all
   2 Just a little bad
   3 Pretty bad
   4 Very bad
   5 Very, very bad
   0 I did not eat too much

6. How bad did you feel that you could not stop eating or could not control what or how much you were eating?
   1 Not bad at all
   2 Just a little bad
   3 Pretty bad
   4 Very bad
   5 Very, very bad
   0 I did not lose control over my eating

7. During the past 6 months, has your weight or the shape of your body mattered to how you feel about yourself? Compare this feeling to how you feel about other parts of your life – like how you get along with your parents, how you get along with friends, and how you do at school.
   1 Weight and shape were *not important at all* to how I felt about myself.
   2 Weight and shape were *somewhat important* to how I felt about myself.

3 Weight and shape were *pretty important* to how I felt about myself.
4 Weight and shape were *very important* to how I felt about myself.

8. Did you ever *make* yourself vomit, throw up, or get sick to keep from gaining weight after eating a *really big* amount of food?
   1 YES   2 NO   (IF NO: Go to question #9)
   How often – on the average – did you do that?
   1 Less than once a week
   2 Once a week
   3 Two or three times a week
   4 Four or five times a week
   5 More than five times a week

9. Have you ever taken medicine (pills, liquid, gum, powder) that would *make you go to the bathroom* in order to *not gain weight* after eating a *really big* amount of food?
   1 YES   2 NO   (IF NO: Go to question #10)
   Were these laxatives (makes you have a bowel movement or B.M.) or diuretics (makes you urinate or pee)?
   Circle which one(s):   Laxatives   Diuretics
   Did you ever take *more than twice* the amount you were told to take on the box or bottle?
   1 YES   2 NO
   How often – on the average – did you do that?
   1 Less than once a week
   2 Once a week
   3 Two or three times a week
   4 Four or five times a week
   5 More than five times a week

10. Did you ever *not eat anything at all* for at least *24 hours* (a full day) to keep from gaining weight after eating a *really big* amount of food?
    1 YES   2 NO   (IF NO: Go to question #11)
    How often – on the average – did you do that?
    1 Less than once a week
    2 Once a week
    3 Two or three times a week
    4 Four or five tunes a week
    5 More than five times a week

11. Did you ever exercise *for more than one hour* at a time *only* to keep from gaining weight after eating a *really big* amount of food?
    1 YES   2 NO   (IF NO: Go to question #12)
    How often – on the average – did you do that?
    1 Less than once a week
    2 Once a week
    3 Two or three times a week
    4 Four or five times a week
    5 More than five times a week

12. During the past 3 months, did you ever take diet pills to keep from gaining weight after eating a *really big* amount of food?
    1 YES   2 NO   (IF NO: Go on to the next page.)
    Did you ever take more than twice the amount you were told to take on the box or bottle?
    1 YES   2 NO
    How often – on the average – did you do that?
    1 Less than once a week
    2 Once a week
    3 Two or three times a week
    4 Four or five times a week
    5 More than five times a week

Adolescent Version: Parent-Report

1. During the past 6 months, did your child ever eat what most people, like his/her friends, would think was a *really big* amount of food?
   1 YES   2 NO   (IF NO: Go to question #5)
   Did your child every eat a *really big* amount of food within a short time (2 hours or less)?
   1 YES   2 NO   (IF NO: Go to question #5)

2. When your child ate a *really big* amount of food, did you have the impression that he/she could not stop eating or that he/she could not control what or how much he/she was eating?
   1 YES   2 NO   (IF NO: Go to question #5)

3. During the past 6 months, how often did your child eat a *really big* amount of food when you had the impression that his/her eating was out of control?
   There may have been some weeks when your child did not eat this way at all. And some weeks your child may have eaten like this a lot. But, *in general*, how often did this happen?
   1   Less than 1 day a week
   2   One day a week
   3   Two or three days a week
   4   Four or five days a week
   5   Almost every day

4. When your child ate a *really big* amount of food and you thought that he/she could not control his/her eating, did your child:
   a) Eat *very fast*?   Yes   No
   b) Eat until his/her stomach hurt or he/she felt
      sick in the stomach?   Yes   No
   c) Eat *really big* amounts of food even when
      he/she was not hungry?   Yes   No
   d) Eat *really big* amount of food during the day
      without regular meals like breakfast, lunch,
      dinner?   Yes   No
   e) Eat by himself/herself because your child did
      not want anyone to see how much he/she ate?   Yes   No
   f) Feel *really bad* about himself/herself after eating
      a lot of food?   Yes   No

5. During the past 6 months, did you have the impression that your child felt badly when he/she ate too much or more food than he/she thought was best for him/her?
   1   Not at all
   2   Just a little
   3   Pretty much
   4   Very much
   5   Very, very much
   0   My child did not eat too much.

6. How bad did your child feel that he/she could not stop eating or could not control what or how much he/she was eating?
   1   Not at all
   2   Just a little
   3   Pretty much
   4   Very much
   5   Very, very much
   0   My child did not lose control over his/her eating

7. During the past 6 months, did you have the impression that your child's weight or body shape mattered to how your child feels about himself/herself? Compare this feeling to how your child feels about other parts of his/her life – like how he/she gets along with parents, how he/she gets along with friends, and how he/she does at school.
   1   Weight and shape were *not important at all* to how my child felt about himself/herself.

2   Weight and shape were *somewhat important* to how my child felt about himself/herself.
3   Weight and shape were *pretty important* to how my child felt about himself/herself.
4   Weight and shape were *very important* to how my child felt about himself/herself.

8. Did your child ever *make* himself/herself vomit, throw up, or get sick to keep from gaining weight after eating a *really big* amount of food?
   1 YES   2 NO   (IF NO: Go to question #9)
   How often – on the average – did your child do that?
   1   Less than once a week
   2   Once a week
   3   Two or three times a week
   4   Four or five times a week
   5   More than five times a week

9. Has your child ever taken medicine (pills, liquid, gum, powder) that would *make him/her go to the bathroom* in order to *not gain weight* after eating a *really big* amount of food?
   1 YES   2 NO   (IF NO: Go to question #10)
   Were these *laxatives* (makes him/her have a bowel movement) or *diuretics* (Makes him/her urinate or pee)?
   Circle which one(s):   Laxatives   Diuretics
   Did your child ever take *more than twice* the amount he/she was told to take on the box or bottle?
   1 YES   2 NO
   How often – on the average – did your child do that?
   1   Less than once a week
   2   Once a week
   3   Two or three times a week
   4   Four or five times a week
   5   More than five times a week

10. Did your child ever *not eat anything at all* for at least *24 hours* (a full day) to keep from gaining weight after eating a *really big* amount of food?
   1 YES   2 NO   (IF NO: Go to question #11)
   How often – on the average – did your child do that?
   1   Less than once a week
   2   Once a week
   3   Two or three times a week
   4   Four or five times a week
   5   More than five times a week

11. Did your child ever exercise for *more than one hour* at a time *only* to keep from gaining weight after eating a *really big* amount of food?
   1 YES   2 NO   (IF NO: Go to question #12)
   How often – on the average – did your child do that?
   1   Less than once a week
   2   Once a week
   3   Two or three times a week
   4   Four or five times a week
   5   More than five times a week

12. During the past 3 months, did your child ever take diet pills to keep from gaining weight after eating a *really big* amount of food?
   1 YES   2 NO   (IF NO: Stop here)
   Did your child ever take *more than twice* the amount he/she was told to take on the box or bottle?
   1 YES   2 NO
   How often – on the average – did your child do that?
   1   Less than once a week
   2   Once a week
   3   Two or three times a week
   4   Four or five times a week
   5   More than five times a week

3.6 Tics

Motor Tic, Obsessions and Compulsions, Vocal Tic Evaluation Survey (MOVES)

Time 5 minutes.

Ages 7–20

Time Frame Last week

Purpose Assessment of tics.

Commentary

The MOVES was designed to be a brief self-report to assess tics apparent in Tourette's disorder.

Versions

The Motor tic, Obsessions and compulsions, Vocal tic Evaluation Survey (MOVES) is only available as a self-report.

Properties

Items The MOVES comprises 20 items of which 16 basic items pertain to motor and vocal tics, obsessions and compulsions and 4 additional items to associated symptoms. All items are rated on a 4-point scale with responses: never, sometimes, often, and always.

Scales The items of the MOVES are scored on five subscales: Motor Tic, Vocal Tic, Obsessions, Compulsions, and Associated Symptoms. The first two subscales can be combined into the Tic subscale, and the next two subscales can be combined into the OCD subscale. In addition, two total scores can be obtained by summing the 16 basic items and by summing all 20 items.

Reliability Test–retest correlation across a 2-week interval were 0.54 for the Tic subscale, 0.72 for the OCD subscale, and 0.69 for the total score in a patient sample.

Split-half reliability was 0.87 for the 20 items in a patient sample.

Validity The Tic subscale correlated 0.73 with clinician-reported tics, the Obsessions subscale 0.49 with clinician-reported obsessions, the Compulsions subscale with 0.60 clinician-reported compulsions, and the OCD subscale 0.60 with clinician-reported obsessions and compulsions in a patient sample.

The Tic and OCD subscale scores and the total score were significantly higher for patients with Tourette's disorder than for two control groups consisting of patients without tics, obsessions or compulsions, and non-referred subjects. A cut-off score of 10 distinguished the Tourette's disorder group from the control groups with a sensitivity of 0.87 and a specificity of 0.94.

Norms No information available.

Use The MOVES is printed in Gaffney et al. (1994).

Key references

Gaffney GR, Sieg K, Hellings J. The MOVES: A self-rating scale for Tourette's syndrome. J Child Adolesc Psychopharmacol 1994; 4: 269–80.

Address

Gary R. Gaffney
Department of Psychiatry
The University of Iowa Hospitals and Clinics
200 Hawkins Drive, 2880 JPP
Iowa City, Iowa 52242–1009
USA
gary-gaffney@uiowa.edu

Tourette's Disorder Scale (TODS)

Time 5 minutes

Ages 6–17

Time Frame Last week

Purpose Assessment of tics and comorbid symptoms.

Commentary

The TODS was designed as a short and simple instrument to assess overall illness severity of Tourette's disorder. It measures a broad range of common symptoms, including tics, inattention, hyperactivity, obsessions, compulsions, aggression, and emotional symptoms.

Versions

The Tourette's Disorder Scale (TODS) is available in two versions, one rated by parents (TODS-PR) and the other rated by clinicians (TODS-CR).

Properties

Items   The TODS comprises 15 items that are rated on a 11-point scale, of which only 5 responses are labeled: not at all, a little, moderately, markedly, and extremely.

Scales   Factor analysis supported four factors, although item composition of the factors differs somewhat across studies. Subscales based on these factors are labeled: Aggression, ADHD, OCD, and Tics. In addition to the subscales, a total score can be computed as the sum of all items.

Reliability   Interrater correlations ranged from 0.70 to 0.94 for the TODS-CR total score.

Cronbach's alphas were 0.91 and 0.92 for the TODS-PR total score and 0.93 for the TODS-CR total score, and ranged from 0.64 to 0.91 for the subscales of the TODS-PR in clinical children.

Validity   The items correlated significantly with corresponding scales of parent-rated and clinician-rated instruments. The TODS-PR total score, Aggression, ADHD, and OCD correlated significantly with clinician-rated severity of psychopathology and obsessive and compulsive behavior. The TODS-PR total score, Aggression, and OCD correlated significantly with parent-reported depressive symptoms. The TODS-PR Tics score correlated significantly with clinician-rated severity of psychopathology.

The TODS-CR discriminated responders from nonresponders in a clinical trial.

Norms   No information available.

Use   The TODS is printed in Shytle et al. (2003).

Key references

Shytle RD, Silver AA, Sheehan KH, et al. The Tourette's Disorder Scale (TODS): Development, reliability, and validity. Assessment 2003; 10: 273–87.

Storch EA, Murphy TK, Geffken GR, et al. Further psychometric properties of the Tourette's Disorder Scale-Parent rated version (TODS-PR). Child Psychiatr Hum Develop 2004; 35: 107–20.

Address

Doug Shytle
Center for Infant and Child Development
Department of Psychiatry and Behavioral Development, MDC-14
University of South Florida College of Medicine
Tampa, FL 33613
USA
dshytle@hsc.usf.edu

Tourette's Disorder Scale (TODS)

Rated by:

Clinician   Parent

IN THE PAST WEEK, how much has this patient been bothered by the following symptoms?

	Not at all		A little			Moderately			Markedly		Extremely	
1	0	1	2	3	4	5	6	7	8	9	10	Irritable
2	0	1	2	3	4	5	6	7	8	9	10	Motor tics
3	0	1	2	3	4	5	6	7	8	9	10	Argumentative
4	0	1	2	3	4	5	6	7	8	9	10	Sudden mood changes
5	0	1	2	3	4	5	6	7	8	9	10	Demands attention
6	0	1	2	3	4	5	6	7	8	9	10	Hot temper
7	0	1	2	3	4	5	6	7	8	9	10	Vocal tics
8	0	1	2	3	4	5	6	7	8	9	10	Obsessions*
9	0	1	2	3	4	5	6	7	8	9	10	Inattention
10	0	1	2	3	4	5	6	7	8	9	10	Loud/talkative
11	0	1	2	3	4	5	6	7	8	9	10	Restless
12	0	1	2	3	4	5	6	7	8	9	10	Compulsions*
13	0	1	2	3	4	5	6	7	8	9	10	Tense, anxious, nervous
14	0	1	2	3	4	5	6	7	8	9	10	Depressed or uninterested in most things
15	0	1	2	3	4	5	6	7	8	9	10	Impulsive

Obsessions*

In the past week, has the patient been bothered by recurrent unwanted thoughts that kept coming into his/her mind that (s)he couldn't get rid of: like bad thoughts or urges; or nasty pictures? For example, did (s)he think about hurting somebody even though (s)he knew (s)he didn't want to? Was (s)he afraid (s)he or someone would get hurt because of some little thing (s)he did or didn't do? Was (s)he afraid that (s)he would do something really shocking? Does (s)he feel that things need to be 'just right'.

(NOTE: DO NOT INCLUDE SIMPLE EXCESSIVE WORRIES ABOUT REAL LIFE PROBLEMS. DO NOT INCLUDE OBSESSIONS DIRECTLY RELATED TO EATING DISORDERS, SEXUAL BEHAVIOR, OR ALCOHOL OR DRUG ABUSE BECAUSE THE PATIENT MAY DERIVE PLEASURE FROM THE ACTIVITY AND MAY WANT TO RESIST IT ONLY BECAUSE OF ITS NEGATIVE CONSEQUENCES)

Compulsions*

In the past week, has the patient performed tasks or certain acts over and over without being able to stop doing it, like checking, counting, touching, washing, or organizing things over and over; or saying or doing something over and over until it feels 'just right'.

Yale Global Tic Severity Scale (YGTSS)

Time 10 minutes

Ages 5–51

Time Frame Last week

Purpose Assessment of tics.

Commentary

The YGTSS was designed for the use of experienced clinicians following the completion of a semi-structured interview with multiple informants.

Versions

The Yale Global Tic Severity Scale (YGTSS) is only available as a clinician report.

Properties

Items   The YGTSS comprises 10 items pertaining to number, frequency, intensity, complexity, and interference of motor and phonic tics, and 1 item indicating overall impairment of tic symptoms. The items are rated on a 6-point scale with different descriptions of response options across items.

Scales   The items pertaining to the tic ratings are scored on two subscales, which are supported by factor analysis. The subscales are: Motor Tics, and Phonic Tics. In addition, the Global Severity Score is the sum of the two subscales and the item indicating overall impairment.

Reliability   Interrater intraclass correlations among three raters ranged from 0.52 to 0.99 for the motor tic items, from 0.67 to 0.82 for the phonic tic items, and were 0.78 for Motor Tics, 0.91 for Phonic Tic, 0.80 for overall impairment, and 0.85 for Global Severity Score.

Validity   The subscales Motor Tics and Phonic Tics and the Global Severity Score correlated 0.86, 0.91, and 0.62, respectively with comparable subscales from another clinician-rated scale for assessing tics.

The Global Severity Score correlated 0.82, 0.11, 0.39, and –0.36 with clinician-reported tic, ADHD, OCD, and positive scaled global impairment, respectively.

Norms   No information available.

Use   An instructional manual describing the YTGSS and its administration is available from James F. Leckman at the address below.

Key references

Leckman JF, Riddle MA, Hardin MT, et al. The Yale Gobal Tic Severity Scale: Initial testing of a clinician-rated scale of tic severity. J Am Acad Child Adolesc Psychiatry 1989; 28: 566–73.

Address

James F. Leckman
Child Study Center
Yale University School of Medicine
230 South Frontage Rd.
New Haven, CT 06520–7900
USA
james.leckman@yale.edu

Yale Global Tic Severity Scale (YGTSS)

A. *Instructions*

This clinical rating scale is designed to rate the overall severity of tic symptoms across a range of dimensions (number, frequency, intensity, complexity, and interference). Use of the YGTSS requires the rater to have clinical experience with Tourette's syndrome patients. The final rating is based on all available information and reflects the clinician's overall impression for each of the items to be rated.

The style of the interview is semistructured. The interviewer should first complete the Tic Inventory (a list of motor and phonic tics present during the past week, as reported by the parent/patient, and observed during the evaluation). It is then best to proceed with questions based on each of the individual items, using the content of the anchor points as a guide.

B. *Tic Inventory*

1. *Description of Motor Tics:* (Check motor tics present during past week)

   a. *Simple Motor Tics:* (Rapid, Darting, 'Meaningless'):
   _____ Eye blinking
   _____ Eye movements
   _____ Nose movements
   _____ Mouth movements
   _____ Facial grimace
   _____ Head jerks/movements
   _____ Shoulder shrugs
   _____ Arm movements
   _____ Band movements
   _____ Abdominal tensing
   _____ Leg or foot or toe movements
   _____ Other _____
   _____
   _____

   b. *Complex Motor Tics:* (Slower, 'Purposeful'):
   _____ Eye gestures or movements
   _____ Mouth movements
   _____ Facial movements or expressions
   _____ Head gestures or movements
   _____ Shoulder gestures
   _____ Arm or hand gestures
   _____ Writing tics
   _____ Dystonic postures
   _____ Bending or gyrating
   _____ Rotating
   _____ Leg or foot or toe movements
   _____ Tic-related compulsive behaviors (touching, tapping, grooming, evening-up)
   _____ Copropraxia
   _____ Self abusive behavior (describe) _____
   _____
   _____ Paroxysms of tics (displays), duration _____ seconds
   _____ Disinhibited behavior (describe)* _____
   _____
   _____ Other _____
   _____
   _____ Describe any orchestrated patterns or sequences of motor tic behaviors _____
   _____

2. *Description of Phonic Tic Symptoms:* (Check phonic tics present over the past week)

   a. *Simple Phonic Symptoms:* (Fast, 'Meaningless' Sounds):

Sounds, noises; (circle: coughing, throat clearing, sniffing, grunting, whistling, animal or bird noises)
Other (list) _____
_____

b. *Complex Phonic Symptoms:* (Language: Words, Phrases, Statements):
_____ Syllables: (list) _____
_____ Words: (list) _____
_____ Coprolalia: (list) _____
_____ Echolalia _____
_____ Palalali _____
_____ Blocking _____
_____ Speech atypicalities: (describe). _____
_____ Disinhibited speech: (describe)*. _____
_____ Describe any orchestrated patterns or sequences of phonic tic behaviors _____

C. *Ordinal Scales* (Rate motor and phonic tics separately unless otherwise indicated).

a. Number: Motor Score: [ ]   Phonic Score: [ ]

Score   Description (Anchor Point)

0   None
1   Single tic
2   Multiple discrete tics (2–5)
3   Multiple discrete tics (>5)
4   Multiple discrete tics plus at least one orchestrated pattern of multiple simultaneous or sequential tics where it is difficult to distinguish discrete tics.
5   Multiple discrete tics plus several (>2) orchestrated patterns of multiple simultaneous or sequential tics where it is difficult to distinguish discrete tics.

b. Frequency: Motor Score: [ ]   Phonic Score: [ ]

Score   Description (Anchor Point)

0   *None.* No evidence of specific tic behaviors.
1   *Rarely.* Specific tic behaviors have been present during previous week. These behaviors occur infrequently, often not on a daily basis. If bouts of tics occur, they are brief and uncommon.
2   *Occasionally.* Specific tic behaviors are usually present on a daily basis, but there are long tic-free intervals during the day. Bouts of tics may occur on occasion and are not sustained for more than a few minutes at a time.
3   *Frequently.* Specific tic behaviors are present on a daily basis. Tic free intervals as long as 3 hours are not uncommon. Bouts of tics occur regularly but may be limited to a single setting.
4   *Almost Always.* Specific tic behaviors are present virtually every waking hour of every day, and periods of sustained tic behaviors occur regularly. Bouts of tics are common and are not limited to a single setting.
5   *Always.* Specific tic behaviors are present virtually all the time. Tic-free intervals are difficult to identify and do not last more than 5 to 10 minutes at most.

c. Intensity   Motor Score: [ ]   Phonic Score: [ ]

Score   Description (Anchor Point)

0   *Absent*
1   *Minimal intensity,* tics not visible or audible (based solely • on patient's private experience) or tics are less forceful than comparable voluntary actions and are typically not noticed because of their intensity.
2   *Mild intensity,* tics are not more forceful than comparable voluntary actions or utterances and are typically not noticed because of their intensity.
3   *Moderate intensity,* tics are more forceful than comparable voluntary actions but are not outside the

---

*Do not include this item in rating the ordinal scales.

range of normal expression for comparable voluntary actions or utterances. They may call attention to the individual because of their forceful character.

4   *Marked intensity,* tics are more forceful than comparable voluntary actions or utterances and typically have an 'exaggerated' character. Such tics frequently call attention to the individual because of their forceful and exaggerated character.

5   *Severe intensity,* tics are extremely forceful and exaggerated in expression. These tics call attention to the individual and may result in risk of physical injury (accidental, provoked, or self-inflicted) because of their forceful expression.

d. *Complexity:*   Motor Score: [   ] Phonic Score: [   ]

Score   Description (Anchor Point)

0   *None,* if present, all tics are clearly 'simple' (sudden, brief, purposeless) in character.

1   *Borderline,* some tics are not clearly 'simple' in character.

2   *Mild,* some tics are clearly 'complex' (purposive in appearance) and mimic brief 'automatic' behaviors, such as grooming, syllables or brief meaningful utterances such as 'ah huh,' 'hi,' that could be readily camouflaged.

3   *Moderate,* some tics are more 'complex' (more purposive and sustained in appearance) and may occur in orchestrated bouts that would be difficult to camouflage but could be rationalized or 'explained' as normal behavior or speech (picking, tapping, saying 'you bet' or 'honey,' brief echolalia).

4   *Marked,* some tics are very 'complex' in character and tend to occur in sustained orchestrated bouts that would be difficult to camouflage and could not be easily rationalized as normal behavior or speech because of their duration and/or their unusual, inappropriate, bizarre, or obscene character (a lengthy facial contortion, touching genitals, echolalia, speech atypicalities, longer bouts of saying 'what do you mean' repeatedly, or saying 'fu' or 'sh').

5   *Severe,* some tics involve lengthy bouts of orchestrated behavior or speech that would be impossible to camouflage or successfully rationalize as normal because of their duration and/or extremely unusual, inappropriate, bizarre, or obscene character (lengthy displays or utterances often involving copropraxia, self-abusive behavior, or coprolalia).

e. *Interference:*   Motor Score: [   ] Phonic Score; [   ]

Score   Description (Anchor Point)

0   *None*

1   *Minimal,* when tics are present, they do not interrupt the flow of behavior or speech.

2   *Mild,* when tics are present, they occasionally interrupt the flow of behavior or speech.

3   *Moderate,* when tics are present, they frequently interrupt the flow of behavior or speech.

4   *Marked,* when tics are present, they frequently interrupt the flow of behavior or speech, and they occasionally disrupt intended action or communication.

5   *Severe,* when tics are present, they frequently disrupt intended action or communication.

f. *Impairment*   Overall Impairment; [   ] (Rate Overall Impairment for Motor and Phonic Tics);

Score   Description (Anchor Point)

0   *None*

10   *Minimal,* tics associated with subtle difficulties in self-esteem, family life, social acceptance, or school or job functioning (infrequent upset or concern about tics vis a vis the future; periodic, slight increase in family tensions because of tics; friends or acquaintances may occasionally notice or comment about tics in an upsetting way).

20   *Mild,* tics associated with minor difficulties in self-esteem, family life, social acceptance, or school or job functioning.

30   *Moderate,* tics associated with some clear problems in self-esteem, family life, social acceptance, or school or job functioning (episodes of dysphoria, periodic distress and upheaval in the family, frequent teasing by peers or epidodic social avoidance, periodic interference in school or job performance because of tics).

40   *Marked,* tics associated with major difficulties in self-esteem, family life, social acceptance, or school or job functioning.

50   *Severe,* tics associated with extreme difficulties in self-esteem, family life, social acceptance, or school or job functioning (sever depression with suicidal ideation, disruption of the family [separation/divorce, residential placement], disruption of social ties – severely restricted life because of social stigma and social avoidance, removal from school or loss of job).

D.   *Score Sheet*

Name _____   Date _____

DOB_____   Sex _____

Sources of Information. _____

_____

_____

Raters   _____

Motor Tics:

Number	[	]
Frequency	[	]
Intensity	[	]
Complexity	[	]
Interference	[	]
Total Motor Tic Score	[	]

Phonic Tics:

Number	[	]
Frequency	[	]
Intensity	[	]
Complexity	[	]
Interference	[	]
Total Phonic Tic Score	[	]
Overall Impairment Rating	[	]
Global Severity Score (Motor + Phonic + Impairment)	[	]

3.7 Developmental Disorders

Asperger Syndrome Diagnostic Scale (ASDS)

Time 10–15 minutes

Ages 5–18

Time Frame Not specified

Purpose Assessment of behaviors associated with Asperger syndrome.

Commentary

The items of the ASDS are based on the DSM-IV and ICD-10 diagnostic criteria of Asperger syndrome (AS) and on a review of literature about AS. The ASDS can be used to identify children who have AS, document progress as a consequence of intervention programs, target goals for change and intervention, and measure AS in research progress.

Versions

The Asperger Syndrome Diagnostic Scale (ASDS) can be completed by parents, teachers or others who have knowledge of a child or are able to observe a child.

Properties

Items   The ASDS comprises 50 items that are rated on a 2-point scale with responses: observed, and not observed. In addition, it comprises 10 open-ended questions on, for example, age of onset of unusual behavior, most problematic behaviors, and settings in which behaviors occur.

Scales   The 50 items are scored on the Asperger Syndrome Quotient (AQS) which is a simple sum of all ratings. In addition, the items are scored on 5 subscales which are labeled: Language, Social, Maladaptive, Cognitive, and Sensorimotor.

Reliability   Cronbach's alpha was 0.83 for the ASQ and ranged from 0.64 to 0.83 for the subscales in a sample of 115 children diagnosed with Asperger syndrome.

The interrater correlation between ratings of parents and teachers of 14 children was 0.93.

Validity   The correlation between the ASQ and a measure for assessing autistic behaviors was not significant.

The ASQ scores were significantly higher for 115 children diagnosed with Asperger syndrome (AS) than for 74 children diagnosed with autism, behavior disorders, ADHD, or learning disabilities (non AS). Discriminant analysis revealed that the ASQ correctly classified children in the AS and non AS groups with an 85% accuracy rate.

Norms   The ASDS is standardized on a sample of 115 children diagnosed with Asperger syndrome. The ASQ is converted to a standardized score with mean 100 and standard deviation 15, and the subscale scores are converted to standardized scores with a mean of 10 and a standard deviation of 3. Both the ASQ and subscale scores are converted to percentile ranks as well.

Use   A manual and forms can be obtained from the publisher at the address below. The first page of each form contains sections for scoring and interpreting the ASDS.

Key references

Myles BS, Bock SJ, RL Simpsom. ASDS: Asperger Syndrome Diagnostic Scale Examiner's Manual. Austin: PRO-ED, Inc, 2001.

Address

PRO-ED, Inc.
8700 Shoal Creek Boulevard
Austin, Texas 78757–6897
USA
www.proedinc.com

Asperger Syndrome Diagnostic Scale (ASDS) – sample items

	Observed	Not observed
4. Does not understand subtle jokes (e.g., sarcasm)	I	0
9. Does not respect others' personal space	I	0
6. Appears depressed or has suicidal tendencies	I	0
2. Displays an extreme or obsessive interest in a narrow subject	I	0
2. Frequently stiffens, flinches, or pulls away when hugged	I	0

Note. From Summary/Response Forms, Asperger Syndrome Diagnostic Scale, by Brenda S Myles, Stacey J Block and Richard L Simpson, 2001, Austin, TX: PRO-ED. www.proedinc.com. Copyright 2001 by PRO-ED, Inc. Reprinted with permission.

Autism Behavior Checklist (ABC)

Time 10 minutes

Ages 1 1/2–35

Time Frame Not specified

Purpose Assessment of autistic behaviors.

Commentary

The ABC was designed to identify individuals with autistic behaviors during initial screening. It is part of the ASIEP-2 (Autism Screening Instrument for Educational planning-Second Edition) which also includes subtests for assessing vocal behavior, social interaction, language performance, communicative abilities, and prognosis of learning rate.

Versions

The Autism Behavior Checklist (ABC) consists of one form that can be completed by teachers and parents.

Properties

Items   The ABC comprises 57 items. If an item is true for an individual, the item is rated with a weighted item response. Weights range from 1 to 4.

Scales   The items are scored on 5 subscales which are labeled: Sensory, Relating, Body and Object Use, Language, and Social and Self Help. The subscales could not be supported by factor analysis (Miranda-Linné et al., 2002). In addition, the total score is the sum of all weighted item ratings.

Reliability   Split-half reliability of the total score was 0.87 in a mixed sample of individuals with and without diagnoses.

Validity   Subscale scores and the total scores were significantly different between a group of individuals diagnosed with autistic disorder and groups of individuals who were mentally retarded, individuals who were deaf and blind, individuals who had emotional disturbances, and individuals who had no disabilities.

Norms   The ABC was standardized on 1049 teacher ratings of individuals aged 18 months to 35 years with and without diagnoses.

Use   A manual and rating scales for the ABC, part of the ASIEP-2, are available from the publisher at the address below.

Key references

Krug DA, Arick JR, Almond PJ. Behavior checklist for identifying severely handicapped individuals with high levels of autistic behaviour. J Child Psychol Psychiatry 1980; 21: 221–9.

Krug DA, Arick JR, Almond PJ. ASIEP-2: Autism Screening Instrument for Educational Planning-Second Edition. Examiner's Manual. Austin: PRO-ED, Inc, 1993.

Miranda-Linné FM, Melin L. A factor analytic study of the Autism Behavior Checklist. J Autism Dev Disord 2002; 32: 181–8.

Address

PRO-ED, Inc.
8700 Shoal Creek Boulevard
Austin, Texas 78757–6897
USA
www.proedinc.com

Autism Behavior Checklist (ABC) – sample items

	Sensory	Relating	Body and object use	Language	Social and self help
	1	2	3	4	5
Does not follow simple commands given once (sit down, come here, stand up)				1	
Does not (or did not as a baby) reach out when reached for		2			
Sometimes shows no 'startle response' to a loud noise (may have thought child was deaf)	3				
Walks on toes			2		
Prefers to manipulate and be occupied with inanimate things					

Note. From Record Form, Autism behavior Checklist, by David A Krug, Joel R Arick and Patricia J Almond, 1992, Austin, TX: PRO-ED. www.proedinc.com. Copyright © 1993 by PRO-ED, Inc. Reprinted with permission.

Autism Spectrum Screening Questionnaire (ASSQ)

Time 10 minutes

Ages 6–17

Time Frame Not specified

Purpose Assessment of autistic behaviors.

Commentary

The ASSQ was developed as a screening instrument to be completed by lay informants for autistic disorders in high-functioning children, especially Asperger's disorder. It is not intended for diagnostic purposes, but as a measure for identifying children who need a more comprehensive evaluation.

Versions

The Autism Spectrum Screening Questionnaire (ASSQ) is available as one report which can be completed by parents and teachers.

Properties

Items   The ASSQ comprises 27 items that are rated on a 3-point scale with responses: no, somewhat, and yes.

Scales   The items of the ASSQ are scored on a total score which is the simple sum of all item ratings.

Reliability   Test–retest correlations across a 2-week interval were 0.96 for parent-reported and 0.94 for teacher-reported ASSQ total scores in a sample of clinical children.

Validity   Correlations of the ASSQ with two general measures of psychopathology were 0.75 and 0.58 for parent reports and 0.77 and 0.70 with teacher reports.

The ASSQ scores were significantly different among three groups of children with autism spectrum disorder, attention-deficit and disruptive disorders, and learning disorder. The ASSQ distinguished children with autism spectrum disorder from children with attention-deficit and disruptive disorders, and learning disorder with a sensitivity of 62% and a specificity of 90% for parent reports and with a sensitivity of 70% and a specificity of 91% for teacher reports.

Norms   A table with means and standard deviations of 6,227 parent ratings and 8,771 teacher ratings of children from the Norwegian general population is printed in Posserud et al. (in press).

Use   The ASSQ is printed in Ehlers and Gillberg (1999).

Key references

Ehlers S, Gillberg C. The epidemiology of Asperger syndrome. A total population study. J Child Psychol Psychiatry 1993; 34: 1327–50.

Ehlers S, Gillberg C, Wing L. A screening questionnaire for Asperger syndrome and other high-functioning autism spectrum disorders in school age children. J Autism Dev Disord 1999; 29: 129–41.

Posserud M, Lundervold AJ, Gillberg C. Autistic features in a total population of 7–9–year-old children assessed by the ASSQ (Autism Spectrum Screening Questionnaire). J Child Psychol Psychiatry 2006; 47: 167–75.

Address

Christopher Gillberg
Department of Child and Adolescent Psychiatry
University of Goteborg
Kungsgatan 12
411 19 Göteborg
Sweden
christopher.gillberg@pediat.gu.se

Autism Spectrum Screening Questionnaire (ASSQ)

Name of child _____   Date of Birth _____

Name of rater _____   Date of rating _____

This child stands out as different from other children of his/her age in the following way:

	No	Somewhat	Yes
1. is old-fashioned or precocious	[ ]	[ ]	[ ]
2. is regarded as an 'eccentric professor' by the other children	[ ]	[ ]	[ ]
3. lives somewhat in a world of his/her own with restricted idiosyncratic intellectual interests	[ ]	[ ]	[ ]
4. accumulates facts on certain subjects (good rote memory) but does not really understand the meaning	[ ]	[ ]	[ ]
5. has a literal understanding of ambiguous and metaphorical language	[ ]	[ ]	[ ]
6. has a deviant style of communication with a formal, fussy, old-fashioned or 'robotlike' language	[ ]	[ ]	[ ]
7. invents idiosyncratic words and expressions	[ ]	[ ]	[ ]
8. has a different voice or speech	[ ]	[ ]	[ ]
9. expresses sounds involuntary; clears throat, grunts, smacks, cries or screams	[ ]	[ ]	[ ]
10. is surprisingly good at some things and surprisingly poor at others	[ ]	[ ]	[ ]
11. uses language freely but fails to make adjustment to fit social contexts or the needs of different listeners	[ ]	[ ]	[ ]
12. lacks empathy	[ ]	[ ]	[ ]
13. makes naive and embarrassing remarks	[ ]	[ ]	[ ]
14. has a deviant style of gaze	[ ]	[ ]	[ ]
15. wishes to be sociable but fails to make relationships with peers	[ ]	[ ]	[ ]
16. can be with other children but only on his/her terms	[ ]	[ ]	[ ]
17. lacks best friend	[ ]	[ ]	[ ]
18. lacks common sense	[ ]	[ ]	[ ]
19. is poor at games: no idea of cooperating in a team, scores 'own goals'	[ ]	[ ]	[ ]
20. has clumsy, ill coordinated, ungainly, awkward movements or gestures	[ ]	[ ]	[ ]
21. has involuntary face or body movements	[ ]	[ ]	[ ]
22. has difficulties in completing simple daily activities because of compulsory repetition of certain actions or thoughts	[ ]	[ ]	[ ]
23. has special routines: insists on no change	[ ]	[ ]	[ ]
24. shows idiosyncratic attachment to objects	[ ]	[ ]	[ ]
25. is bullied by other children	[ ]	[ ]	[ ]
26. has markedly unusual facial expression	[ ]	[ ]	[ ]
27. has markedly unusual posture	[ ]	[ ]	[ ]

Specify reasons other than above:

_____

Reproduced from Ehlers S, Gillberg C, Wing L. A screening questionnaire for Asperger syndrome and other high-functioning autism spectrum disorders in school age children. J Autism Dev Disord 1999; 29: 129–41 with kind permission of Springer Science and Business Media.

Behavioral Summarized Evaluation-Revised (BSE-R)

Time 5 minutes

Ages 11/2–12

Time Frame Last 5 days

Purpose Assessment of autistic behavior.

Commentary

The development of the BSE-R started more than twenty years ago and it was intended to assess developmentally disordered children, especially children with autistic disorders. It can be used as an additional instrument next to informant ratings and diagnostic interviews to obtain an overview of children's autistics behaviors. The BSE-R is an expanded and modified version of the scale that was first described by Bartélémy in1990.

Versions

The Behavioral Summarized Evaluation-Revised (BSE-R) is intended to be completed by raters who observed children during 5 days.

Properties

Items   The BSE-R comprises 29 items that are rated on a 5-point scale with responses: never, sometimes, often, very often, and always. The BSE-R also contains a glossary that gives additional information on how to rate each item.

Scales   Factor analysis was used to determine the structure of the BSE-R. The items are scored on two subscales which are labeled: Interaction Disorder, and Modulation Disorder. In addition, a global score can be obtained by summing all item ratings.

Reliability   The interrater intraclass correlation of the global score between two raters was 0.97 among clinical children.

Validity   Interaction Disorder correlated significantly, but Modulation Disorder not, with parent-reported autistic behavior.

The mean Interaction Disorder score was significantly different among three diagnostic groups of children. Those diagnosed with autistic disorder had significantly higher scores than those diagnosed with mental retardation. Children diagnosed with PDD NOS had significantly lower scores than the children in the other groups. The mean Modulation Disorder score was not significantly different among the three diagnostic groups. The Interaction Disorder scale discriminated between children diagnosed with autistic disorder and children diagnosed with mental retardation or PDD NOS with a sensitivity of 0.74 and a specificity of 0.71.

Norms   An optimal cut point for the classification of autistic disorder among clinical children are given in Barthélémy et al. (1997).

Use   A copy of the BSE-R can be obtained from Catherine Barthélémy at the address below.

Key references

Barthélémy C, Adrien JL, Tanguay P, et al. The Behavior Summarized Evaluation: Validity and reliability of a scale for the assessment of autistic behaviors. J Autism Dev Disord 1990; 20: 189–204.

Barthélémy C, Roux S, Adrien JL, et al. Validation of the revised Behavior Summarized Evaluation scale. J Autism Dev Disord 1997; 27: 139–53.

Address

Catherine Barthélémy
Service Universitaire d'Explorations Fonctionnelles et Neurophysiologie en Pédopsychiatrie
INSERM U 619 (Équipe 1)
CHRU Bretonneau
37 044 Tours Cedex 9
France
catherine.barthelemy@chu-tours.fr

Behavioral Summarized Evaluation-Revised (BSE-R)

The BSE-R Scale is designed to provide a quantitative evaluation of autistic behavior in developmentally disordered children. Each item is scored from 0 to 4 according to the frequency of appearance.

0 = Never
1 = Sometimes
2 = Often
3 = Very often
4 = Always

A cross should be put against the estimated score for each symptom in the column opposite.

No	Item	0	1	2	3	4
1	Aloneness (ALO)	☐	☐	☐	☐	☐
2	Ignores people (IGN)	☐	☐	☐	☐	☐
3	Poor social interaction (SOC)	☐	☐	☐	☐	☐
4	Abnormal eye contact (GAZ)	☐	☐	☐	☐	☐
5	Does not make an effort to communicate using voice and/or words (VOI)	☐	☐	☐	☐	☐
6	Lack of appropriate facial expression and gestures (GES)	☐	☐	☐	☐	☐
7	Stereotyped vocal or verbal utterances, echolalia (ECH)	☐	☐	☐	☐	☐
8	Lack of initiative, poor activity (ACT)	☐	☐	☐	☐	☐
9	Inappropriate relating to inanimate objects or to doll (OBJ)	☐	☐	☐	☐	☐
10	Irresistible and/or ritual use of objects (RIT)	☐	☐	☐	☐	☐
11	Intolerance of change and to frustration (SAM)	☐	☐	☐	☐	☐
12	Stereotyped sensorimotor activity (STE)	☐	☐	☐	☐	☐
13	Agitation, restlessness (AGI)	☐	☐	☐	☐	☐
14	Bizarre posture and gait (POS)	☐	☐	☐	☐	☐
15	Auto-aggressiveness (AGR)	☐	☐	☐	☐	☐
16	Hetero-aggressiveness (HGR)	☐	☐	☐	☐	☐
17	Mild anxiety signs (ANX)	☐	☐	☐	☐	☐
18	Mood difficulties (MOO)	☐	☐	☐	☐	☐
19	Disturbance of feeding behaviour (EAT)	☐	☐	☐	☐	☐
20	Does not try to be clean (stools or urine), plays with stools (CLE)	☐	☐	☐	☐	☐
21	Individual bodily activities (BOD)	☐	☐	☐	☐	☐
22	Sleep problems (SLEP)	☐	☐	☐	☐	☐
23	Unstable attention, easily distracted (ATT)	☐	☐	☐	☐	☐
24	Bizarre responses to auditory stimuli (AUD)	☐	☐	☐	☐	☐
25	Variability (VAR)	☐	☐	☐	☐	☐
26	Does not imitate the gestures and voices of others (IMI)	☐	☐	☐	☐	☐
27	Child too floppy, lifeless (TON)	☐	☐	☐	☐	☐
28	Does not share emotion (EMO)	☐	☐	☐	☐	☐
29	Paradoxical sensitivity to touching and contact (TOU)	☐	☐	☐	☐	☐

1. **Aloneness (ALO)**
   Keeps to the edges of a group or isolates himself/herself from it; cuts off communication.
   Keeps in his/her own world.
   Seeks a familiar space.

2. **Ignores people (IGN)**
   Indifferent to others. Pays no attention to them: can walk into them without seeing them; seems not to hear them.
   Does not respond to overtures.
   Too quiet, indifferent (frozen expression).
   In terms of general behavior there is a turning away from others or a delayed reaction to them.

3. **Poor social interaction (SOC)**
   No exchange of toys.
   No spontaneous approaches; no offering of objects.
   Does not use objects as a means of mediation.
   Uses the adult as an object.
   Does not smile; does not seek company.
   Is incapable of sustaining social exchanges.
   It should be noted that the child can stare at parts of the examiner's body or follow him around and still remain withdrawn.

4. **Abnormal eye contact (GAZ)**
   Does not look you in the eye; covers eyes; avoids direct looks.
   Looks away; turns face away when called or looked at.
   Empty or lifeless expression; fleeting or piercing look; follows things with eyes only intermittently; fixes things with gaze peripherally rather than centrally.

5. **Does not make an effort to communicate using voice and/or words (VOI)**
Here assessment should be based on the effort towards communication and not on verbal level. A child with speech can make no effort to communicate and score a high mark (noncommunicative echolalic language). A child without speech can try to make himself/herself understood in his/her own way (burbling, prattling) and score a low mark.

6. **Lack of appropriate facial expression and gestures (GES)**
Amimia. Facial immobility.
Shows no anticipatory postural reaction when about to be picked up.
Cannot direct the examiner's hand to obtain a desired object: does not wave hands in its direction: cannot indicate precisely what s/he wants by gesture, attitude, or look.
If s/he can speak, does not use facial, vocal, or gestural expression with normal frequency and liveliness.

7. **Stereotyped vocal or verbal utterances, echolalia (ECH)**
Immediate or delayed echolalia; repeats randomly or selectively. Inversion of the personal pronoun.
Repeats words or phrases whether or not they have communicative value.
Links together words and phrases based on certain key words or consonances irrespective of any logical connection between them. Example: lemon, Monday, daylight, etc.
Utters stereotyped sounds ('ah,' 'oh') in an abrupt, jerky way at moments of disappointment or delight: at other times for no particular reason.

8. **Lack of initiative, poor activity (ACT)**
Does not invent any games without prompting (though possibly quite capable of doing so).
Passivity; lack of interest.
Slowness.

9. **Inappropriate relating to inanimate objects or to doll (OBJ)**
Ignores objects or shows only fleeting interest in them (the object is held in a haphazard way without visual fixation on it).
Sucks or puts objects into mouth.
Pats, taps or strikes them repeatedly.
Unusual behavior towards objects; lets them drop from hands passively: strokes them.
Pulls hand away from a building block as if it were red-hot: minute tactile examination of things; tends to become absorbed by meaningless marks: stains, holes, dots.
Bizarre and very personal utilization of objects and/or strange, eccentric behavior; will place an object on its side, or turn it round and round. Always carries a piece of string. Picks up anything lying around.

10. **Irresistible and/or ritual use of objects (RIT)**
Irresistible, uncontrollable need for an object, always keeps it with him/her, whether or not s/he uses it.
Always uses objects in the same way and for the same purpose.

11. **Intolerance of change and frustration (SAM)**
Insistent demand that everything remains unchanged.
Has great difficulty in accepting anything unusual: changes of place, time, people, clothes, food. Such changes provoke disproportionate reactions.
Frustrated, reacts angrily when forbidden something or when activities are interrupted: discontented when desires or expectations remain unsatisfied. Becomes fixated on the frustrating element.

12. **Stereotyped sensorimotor activity (STE)**
Stereotyped activities can also be noticed in the gait:
Rocks to and fro on the bed, on the ground or from one foot to the other.
Looks at hands; plays 'hand-games', twists fingers, smells hands, blocks ears, covers eyes.
Drums feet.
Plays 'eye-games' in sunlight or electric light.

13. **Agitation, restlessness (AGI)**
Such symptoms occur in periods of rest or directed activity.
Restlessness: disordered, uncontrolled, aimless excitation.
Seems unable to find any peace, is constantly on the move.
Boisterousness: seems compelled to make a noise and be generally troublesome. Boisterousness can be considered normal, but pathological when exaggerated. It is therefore taken into account in the assessment.
Example: climbs everywhere, jumps from chair to chair, touches everything, is constantly changing activities, spreads out objects or toys. Can also be very noisy and deliberately seek out noise 'like a tornado'.

14. **Bizarre posture and gait (POS)**
Strangeness is often evident in posture and gait but it can also extend to general behavior and activities.
Facial expression: grimaces, bizarre facial movements
Posture: feet crossed in the air, head underneath; twisted body; unbalanced posture; legs folded, head against the feet: hunched up in the corner of a room; neck bent backwards; violent extensions of the body; absence of postural anticipation; poor postural adaptation (the 'soft' or 'slippery' child).
Gait: hops, walks on tiptoe or on the heels; turns round and round or runs round in little circles; walks dragging one foot; walks sideways with strange sudden forward movements.

15. **Auto-aggressiveness (AGR)**
Aggression directed against or mutilation of own body (hits head with hand or some object, lets himself/herself fall heavily to the ground, bites, pinces himself/herself, scratches face, etc.).

16. **Heteroaggressiveness (HGR)**
Bites, scratches, hits out at other people.

17. **Mild anxiety signs (ANX)**
Examples of manifestations of anguish and anxiety:
Sudden fits or crying, whimpering (often without tears)
Little nervous laughs
Seems fearful, fretful, uneasy
Aimless walking up and down
Trembling
Somatization: vomiting, hyperventilation or retention of breath, intestinal problems (constipation, diarrhea), sweating, nail-biting.

18. **Mood difficulties (MOO)**
Difficulty in registering emotion
Alternation of opposite emotions (anger, laughter, pleasure, sadness)
Unprovoked fits of temper and laughter.

19. **Disturbance of feeding behavior (EAT)**
Qualitative and/or quantitative difficulties
Passive indifference: allows himself/herself to be fed without affective participation.
Active refusal: cries or screams at the sight of food, refuses to be fed, gesticulating and turning the head away.
Exclusive choice of certain tastes: sweet or salty.
Eats other things (stones, paper).
Coprophagy.
Meryscism: 'ruminates'.
Vomiting.
Eats dirtily, smears the food or throws it away.
Rituals.
Absence of the sense of taste.
Bulimia, anorexia.

20. **Does not try to be clean (stools or urine), plays with stools (CLE)**
It is necessary to appreciate the efforts to be clean and not autonomy which varies with age. Plays with stools, handles them, puts them in mouth.

21. Individual bodily activities (BOD)

Including:

Solitory stimulation of sensitive areas of body, particularly sexual areas (masturbation).

Seeks or avoids 'skin' contact with others: sexual games, problems with bodily contact.

Disinterested in body, no handling of parts of the body (mouth, anus, sexual organs, skin).

The child avoids bodily contact during washing, dressing, etc. Avoids being touched.

22. Sleep problems (SLEP)

Hypersomnia (sleepy, difficult to waken).

Hyposomnia (too awake, active, excitable). The child can remain awake and calm.

Disturbed sleep (screams, cries, complains, nightmares, nightfears).

Sleep rituals (needs a presence, certain positions).

23. Unstable attention, easily distracted (ATT)

The child is incapable of fixing his attention on any suggested activity.

Takes no notice of what is said to him/her on any suggested activity.

Slowness of integration: does not take in instructions or does so only after a delay.

Delayed responses.

Unstable attention: modifications of attention are triggered by minute changes in the environment.

Abnormal attention: pays attention to own nonvocal sound productions (scratching, tapping), which s/he listens to very attentively.

24. Bizarre responses to auditory stimuli (AUD)

Heightened importance of the auditory function in a certain kind of relation with the outside world.

Excessive, insufficient, or selective sensitivity to noises, sounds, calls.

Paradoxical responses. Example: the child does not turn head when a door slams or when his/her name is called and interests himself/herself instead in the sound of rustling paper.

25. Variability (VAR)

Considerable, even extreme, variations in capacities or problems from one minute to another.

These variations may also involve behaviour with others in the form of aggressive rejection or possessive attachment.

26. Does not imitate the gestures or voices of others (IMI)

Incapable of copying movements of hands, head, mouth or of copying postures and does not imitate sounds (not to be confused with echopraxia or echolalia).

27. Child too floppy, lifeless (TON)

Hypotonic child, limp.

28. Does not share emotion (EMO)

Does not seem sensitive to emotion expressed by others. The expression of his/her emotion does not fit with that of others.

29. Paradoxical sensitivity to touching and contact (TOU)

Physical contact with objects or people are sometimes avoided and sometimes accepted, even sought.

Remarks

Certain considerations that could suddenly modify the scores should be clearly indicated: e.g., child changes group or treatment, the nurse or teacher changes etc.

Checklist for Autism in Toddlers (CHAT)

Time 15 minutes

Ages 18 months

Time Frame Not specified

Purpose Assessment of autistic behavior.

Commentary

The CHAT was designed for the early identification of autism in children aged 18 months. Key items of the CHAT focus on two behaviors: 1. joint attention, e.g. looking to where a parent is pointing; 2. pretend play, e.g. pretending to pour tea from a toy teapot. If children are lacking these behaviors at age 18 months, they are at risk for a social-communication disorder.

Versions

The Checklist for Autism in Toddlers (CHAT) is only available as one form that includes questions for both parents and primary health care workers.

Properties

Items   The CHAT comprises 14 items. The first 9 items are asked to the parents, and the last 5 items are made by the primary health care worker. All items are rated on a 2-point scale with responses: yes, and no.

Scales   The items of the CHAT are not scored on subscales. Instead, the CHAT has 5 key items and if children fail on these items they have a high risk of developing autism. Children who fail on 2 specific key items have a medium risk of developing autism.

Reliability   No information available.

Validity   In a population-screening study of 16 000 18-months-old children the CHAT was able to detect children with a diagnosis of autism with a sensitivity of 18% and a specificity of 100%, and to detect children with all pervasive developmental disorders with a sensitivity of 21% and a specificity of 100%.

Norms   No information available.

Use   The CHAT and further information can be downloaded from the website of the Autism Research Centre.

Key references

Baron-Cohen S, Allen J, Gillberg C. Can autism be detected at 18 months? The needle, the haystack, and the CHAT. Br J Psychiatry 1992; 161: 839–43.

Baron-Cohen S, Wheelwright S, Cox A, et al. Psychological markers in the detection of autism in infancy in a large population. Br J Psychiatry 2000; 168: 158–63.

Baron-Cohen S, Cox A, Baird G, et al. Early identification of autism by the Checklist for Autism in Toddlers (CHAT). J R Soc Med 2000; 93: 521–5.

Address

Simon Baron-Cohen
Autism Research Centre (ARC)
Cambridge University
Douglas House
18b Trumpington Road
Cambridge CB2 2AH
UK
sb205@cam.ac.uk
www.autismresearchcentre.com

Checklist for Autism in Toddlers (CHAT)

To be used by GPs or health visitors during the 18-month developmental check-up.

Child's name _____   Date of Birth _____   Age _____

Child's address _____   Phone number _____

Section A. Ask parent:

1.	Does your child enjoy being swung, bounced on your knee, etc?	Yes	No
2.	Does your child take an interest in other children?	Yes	No
3.	Does your child like climbing on things, such as up stairs?	Yes	No
4.	Does your child enjoy playing peek-a-boo/hide-and-seek?	Yes	No
5.	Does your child ever pretend, for example, to make a cup of tea using a toy cup and teapot, or pretend other things?	Yes	No
6.	Does your child ever use his/her index finger to point, to ask for something?	Yes	No
7.	Does your child ever use his/her index finger to point, to indicate interest in something?	Yes	No
8.	Can your child play properly with small toys (e.g. cars or bricks) without just mouthing, fiddling, or dropping them?	Yes	No
9.	Does your child ever bring objects over to you (parent), to show you something?	Yes	No

Section B. GP's or health visitor's observation:

i.	During the appointment, has the child made eye contact with you?	Yes	No
ii.	Get child's attention, then point across the room at an interesting object and say 'Oh look! There's a [name a toy]!' Watch child's face. Does the child look across to see what you are pointing at?	Yes[1]	No
iii.	Get the child's attention, then give child a miniature toy cup and teapot and say 'Can you make a cup of tea?' Does the child pretend to pour out tea, drink it, etc?	Yes[2]	No
iv.	Say to the child 'Where's the light?', or 'Show me the light'. Does the child point with his/her index finger at the light?	Yes[3]	No
v.	Can the child build a tower of bricks? (If so, how many?) (Number of bricks ...)	Yes	No

1. To record yes on this item, ensure the child has not simply looked at your hand, but has actually looked at the object you are pointing at.
2. If you can elicit an example of pretending in some other game, score a yes on this item.
3. Repeat this with 'Where's the teddy?' or some other unreachable object, If child does not understand the word 'light'. To record yes on this item, the child must have looked up at your face around the time of pointing.

© The Royal College of Psychiatrists. Reproduced by permission from Baron-Cohen S, Allen J, Gillberg C (1992) Can autism be detected at 18 months? The needle, the haystack, and the CHAT. British Journal of Psychiatry, 161:839–843.

Childhood Asperger Syndrome Test (CAST)

Time 10–15 minutes

Ages 4–11

Time Frame Not specified

Purpose Assessment of behaviors associated with Asperger syndrome.

Commentary

Autism is now routinely identified by the age of 3 years and can be identified as young as 18 months. However, Asperger syndrome is currently identified around 11 years of age. The CAST was designed to identify children with Asperger syndrome as young as 4 years.

Versions

The Childhood Asperger Syndrome Test (CAST) is only available as a parent-report form.

Properties

Items   The CAST comprises 37 items that are scored on a 2-point scale with responses: yes, and no. In addition, it comprises 7 items pertaining to special needs of children with Asperger syndrome that are rated on the same 2-point scale.

Scales   The items of the CAST are scored on a total score which is the simple sum of the ratings of 31 items assessing behaviors associated with Asperger syndrome.

Reliability   No information available.

Validity   Item responses were significantly different between children diagnosed with Asperger syndrome and normal developing children for all but 4 items and between children divided into AS-cases and non AS-cases based assessments for all but 3 items. A cut-off score of 15 for the total score discriminated between children diagnosed with AS and children without AS based on consensus diagnosis with a sensitivity of 100%, and a sensitivity of 97%.

Norms   A cut-off score of 15 for the total score of the CAST can be used to identify children with Asperger syndrome.

Use   The CAST and scoring instructions can be downloaded from www.autismresearchcentre.com.

Key references

Scott FJ, Baron-Cohen S, Bolton P, Brayne C. The CAST (Childhood Asperger Syndrome Test): Preliminary development of a UK screen for mainstream primary-school-age children. Autism 2002; 6: 9–31.

Williams J, Scott FJ, Stott C, et al. The CAST (Childhood Asperger Syndrome Test): Test accuracy. Autism 2005; 9: 45–68.

Address

Fiona J Scott
Autism Research Centre
Douglas House
University of Cambridge
18b Trumpington Road
Cambridge CB2 2AH
UK
fjs25@cus.cam.ac.uk

Childhood Asperger Syndrome Test (CAST)

Child's name: _____ Age: _____ Sex: male/female

Birth order: _____ Twin or single birth: _____

Parent/guardian: _____

Parent(s) occupation: _____

Age parent(s) left full-time education: _____

Address: _____

Tel. no.: _____ School: _____

Please read the following questions carefully, and circle the appropriate answer. All responses are confidential.

1	Does s/he join in playing games with other children easily?	Yes	No
2	Does s/he come up to you spontaneously for a chat?	Yes	No
3	Was s/he speaking by 2 years old?	Yes	No
4	Does s/he enjoy sports?	Yes	No
5	Is it important to him/her to fit in with the peer group?	Yes	No
6	Does s/he appear to notice unusual details that others miss?	Yes	No
7	Does s/he tend to take things literally?	Yes	No
8	When s/he was 3 years old, did s/he spend a lot of time pretending (e.g. play-acting being a superhero, or holding teddy's tea parties)?	Yes	No
9	Does s/he like to do things over and over again, in the same way all the time?	Yes	No
10	Does s/he find it easy to interact with other children?	Yes	No
11	Can s/he keep a two-way conversation going?	Yes	No
12	Can s/he read appropriately for his/her age?	Yes	No
13	Does s/he mostly have the same interests as his/her peers?	Yes	No
14	Does s/he have an interest which takes up so much time that s/he does little else?	Yes	No
15	Does s/he have friends, rather than just acquaintances?	Yes	No
16	Does s/he often bring you things s/he is interested in to show you?	Yes	No
17	Does s/he enjoy joking around?	Yes	No
18	Does s/he have difficulty understanding the rules for polite behaviour?	Yes	No
19	Does s/he appear to have an unusual memory for details?	Yes	No
20	Is his/her voice unusual (e.g. overly adult, flat, or very monotonous)?	Yes	No
21	Are people important to him/her?	Yes	No
22	Can s/he dress him/herself?	Yes	No
23	Is s/he good at turn-taking in conversation?	Yes	No
24	Does s/he play imaginatively with other children, and engage in role-play?	Yes	No
25	Does s/he often do or say things that are tactless or socially inappropriate?	Yes	No
26	Can s/he count to 50 without leaving out any numbers?	Yes	No
27	Does s/he make normal eye-contact?	Yes	No
28	Does s/he have any unusual and repetitive movements?	Yes	No
29	Is his/her social behaviour very one-sided and always on his/her own terms?	Yes	No
30	Does s/he sometimes say 'you' or 's/he' when s/he means 'I'?	Yes	No
31	Does s/he prefer imaginative activities such as play-acting or story-telling, rather than numbers or lists of facts?	Yes	No
32	Does s/he sometimes lose the listener because of not explaining what s/he is talking about?	Yes	No
33	Can s/he ride a bicycle (even if with stabilizers)?	Yes	No
34	Does s/he try to impose routines on him/herself, or on others, in such a way that it causes problems?	Yes	No
35	Does s/he care how s/he is perceived by the rest of the group?	Yes	No
36	Does s/he often turn conversations to his/her favourite subject rather than following what the other person wants to talk about?	Yes	No
37	Does s/he have odd or unusual phrases?	Yes	No

Special needs section

Please complete as appropriate.

38	Have teachers/health visitors ever expressed any concerns about his/her development? If yes, please specify:..	Yes	No
39	Has s/he ever been diagnosed with any of the following?:		
	Language delay	Yes	No
	Hyperactivity/attention deficit disorder (ADHD)	Yes	No
	Hearing or visual difficulties	Yes	No
	Autism spectrum condition, inc. Asperger syndrome	Yes	No
	A physical disability	Yes	No
	Other (please specify)	Yes	No

Childhood Autism Rating Scale (CARS)

Time 5 minutes

Ages 2 years and older

Time Frame Not specified

Purpose Assessment of autistic behaviors.

Commentary

The CARS was first published in 1971 and was intended to enable clinicians to obtain a more objective diagnosis of autism in a more readily usable form. It was first developed as a research instrument, but was revised to evaluate children who were referred to a program for treatment and education of autistic children.

Versions

The Childhood Autism Rating Scale (CARS) was intended to be completed by clinicians and other professionals, but it can also be rated from medical records, classroom observations, and parent reports.

Properties

Items The CARS comprises 15 items that are rated on a 7-point scale with responses: within normal limits for that age, very mildly abnormal for that age, mildly abnormal for that age, mildly-to-moderately abnormal for that age, moderately abnormal for that age, moderately-to-severely abnormal for that age, and severely abnormal for that age. Four response options have extensive labels, which are shown in the sample items below. Three response options are between these labeled options.

Scales The items of the CARS constitute a total score, which is the sum of all item ratings.

Reliability Test–retest correlation across a 1-year interval was 0.88.

Cronbach's alpha was 0.94 for the total score.

Validity The CARS correlated 0.84 with clinical ratings obtained during the same diagnostic sessions and 0.80 with clinical ratings based on information obtained from referral records, and parent and child interviews.

CARS ratings based on testing sessions did not differ significantly from ratings obtained from parent interviews, from classroom observations, and from case history charts. Correlations were 0.82, 0.73, and 0.82, respectively. CARS ratings did not differ significantly between professionals with extensive experience and professionals who have less experience with autism. The correlation between the two types of professionals was 0.83.

Norms The CARS was standardized on 1606 ratings of children aged 0–18 years referred to a program for treatment and education of autistic children.

Use A manual and rating scales enabling direct scoring are available from the publisher at the address below.

Key references

Schopler E, Reichler RJ, CeVellis RF, Daly K. Toward objective classification of childhood autism: Childhood Autism Rating Scale (CARS). J Autism Dev Disord 1980; 10: 91–103.

Schopler E, Reichler RJ, Rochen Renner B. The Childhood Autism Rating Scale (CARS). Los Angeles: Western Psychological Services, 1988.

Address

Western Psychological Services
12031 Wilshire Blvd.
Los Angeles, CA 90025–1251
USA
www.wpspublish.com

Childhood Autism Rating Scale (CARS) – sample items

III. Emotional response

1 Age-appropriate and situation-appropriate emotional responses. The child shows the appropriate type and degree of emotional response as indicated by a change in facial expression, posture, and manner.

1.5

2 Mildly abnormal emotional responses. The child occasionally displays a somewhat inappropriate type or degree of emotional reactions. Reactions are sometimes unrelated to the objects or events surrounding them.

2.5

3 Moderately abnormal emotional responses. The child shows definite signs of inappropriate type and/or degree of emotional response. Reactions may be quite inhibited or expressive and unrelated to the situation, may grimace, laugh, or become rigid even though no apparent emotion producing objects are present.

3.5

4 Severely abnormal emotional responses. Responses are seldom appropriate to the situation; once the child gets in a certain mood, it is very difficult to change the mood. Conversely, the child may show wildly different emotions when nothing has changed.

Observations:

XI. Verbal communication

1 Normal verbal communication, age and situation appropriate.

1.5

2 Mildly abnormal verbal communication. Speech shows overall retardation. Most speech is meaningful; however, some echolalia or pronoun reversal may occur. Some peculiar words or jargon may be used occasionally.

2.5

3 Moderately abnormal verbal communication. Speech may be absent. When present, verbal communication may be a mixture of some meaningful speech and some peculiar speech such as jargon, echolalia, or pronoun reversal. Peculiarities in meaningful speech include excessive questioning or preoccupation with particular topics.

3.5

4 Severely abnormal verbal communication. Meaningful speech is not used. The child may make infantile squeals, weird or animal-like sounds, complex noises approximating speech, or may show persistent, bizarre use of some recognizable words or phrases.

Observations:

Children's Communication Checklist – Second Edition (CCC-2)

Time 5–15 minutes

Ages 4–16

Time Frame Not specified, although the instruction on the checklist refers to the last week when respondents find it hard to make up their mind.

Purpose Assessment of communication problems.

Commentary

The CCC-2 is under development for 10 years. Its main function is to assess aspects of communication that are not easy to evaluate in more traditional one-to-one clinical assessment. Traditional tests are insensitive to pragmatic communication problems, which are dependent on context. Therefore, the CCC-2 was designed to be completed by an adult who has regular contact with a child. The CCC-2 can assist in identifying children who may merit further assessment for an autistic spectrum disorder.

Versions

The Children's Communication Checklist – Second Edition (CCC-2) is usually completed by a parent, although it can be completed by any adult who has had regular contact with the child for at least 3–4 days per week for at least 3 months. Normative data come from parent-completed checklists.

Properties

Items The CCC-2 comprises 70 items that are rated on a 4-point scale with responses: less than once a week (or never); at least once a week, but not every day; once or twice a day; and several times (more than twice) a day (or always). The CCC-2 starts with items pertaining to difficulties with communication and ends with items pertaining to communicative strengths.

Scales The items of the CCC-2 are scored on 10 subscales of which each comprises 2 items pertaining to communicative strengths and 5 to communicative difficulties. Four subscales assess aspects of language structure: speech, syntax, semantics, and coherence. Four subscales assess pragmatic aspects of communication: inappropriate communication, stereotyped language, use of context, and nonverbal communication. Two subscales assess behaviors pertaining to autistic disorder. In addition, two composite scores can be derived from the subscales. The General Communication Composite (GCC) may be used to identify children with communication problems and the Social Interaction Deviance Composite (SIDC) may be used to identify children with a communication profile characteristic of autism.

Reliability Cronbach's alphas ranged from 0.66 to 0.80 for the subscales in normal children.

Validity Among clinical groups of children diagnosed with specific language impairment, pragmatic language impairment with or without autism, high-functioning autism, Asperger syndrome, and a control group of children with normal development, all subscale scores of the clinical groups were significantly lower than the control group. Children with clinically significant communication disorders are unlikely to score above the 10th percentile on the GCC and the majority score below the 3rd percentile. The SIDC is sensitive in separating communication disorders from autistic spectrum disorders.

Norms The CCC-2 was standardized on 542 parent-completed checklists of children from the general population in the United Kingdom. The raw scores of the subscales are converted to age scaled scores with a mean of 10 and a standard deviation of 3. These age-scaled scores and the GCC are converted to percentiles.

Use A manual, checklists, summary sheets, scoring overlays, and a scoring program can be obtained from the publisher at the address below.

Key references

Bishop DVM. Development of the Children's Communication Checklist (CCC): A method for assessing qualitative aspects of communicative impairment in children. J Child Psychol Psychiatry 1998; 39: 879–91.

Bishop DVM. The Children's Communication Checklist Second Edition: CCC-2 Manual. London: Harcourt Assessment, 2003.

Norbury CF, Hash M, Baird, Bishop DVM. Using a parental checklist to identify diagnostic groups in children with communication impairment: A validation of the Children's Communication Checklist-2. Int J Lang Commun Disord 2004; 39: 345–64.

Address

Harcourt Assessment
Procter House
1 Procter Street
London WC1V 6EU
United Kingdom
www.harcourt-uk.com

Gilliam Asperger's Disorder Scale (GADS)

Time 10 minutes

Ages 3–22

Time Frame Not specified

Purpose Assessment of Asperger's disorder behavior.

Commentary

The GADS was based on the diagnostic criteria for Asperger's disorder in the DSM-IV-TR and the ICD-10.

Versions

The Gilliam Asperger's Disorder Scale (GADS) consists of one form that can be completed by parents and professionals at home and school.

Properties

Items The GADS comprises 32 items assessing observed behaviors that are rated on a 4-point scale with responses: never observed, seldom observed, sometimes observed, and frequently observed. In addition, the GADS comprises 20 items about a child's development before age 3 years that are rated on a 2-point scale with responses: yes, and no. The GADS also comprises several open-ended questions to help examiners reach a conclusion.

Scales The items about observed behaviors of the GADS are scored on four subscales which are labeled: Social Interaction, Restricted Patterns of Behavior, Cognitive Patterns, and Pragmatic Skills. In addition, the Asperger's Disorder Quotient is computed by summing the subscales and converting the sum into a quotient. The yes-no items are not scored on subscales.

Reliability Test–retest correlations across a 2-week interval ranged from 0.71 to 0.77 for the subscales and the correlation was 0.93 for the Asperger's Disorder Quotient in a sample of children with Asperger's disorder.

Cronbach's alphas ranged from 0.70 to 0.90 for the subscales and from 0.88 to 0.95 for the Asperger's Disorder Quotient across several samples.

Validity Correlations between the GADS subscales and corresponding subscales of a parent- and teacher-reported measure of autistic behavior ranged from 0.24 to 0.64, while correlations between non-corresponding subscales ranged from 0.06 to 0.67. Total scores of both measures correlated 0.58.

The subscales scores and the Asperger's Disorder Index were significantly higher in a group of individuals diagnosed with Asperger's disorder than a group of individuals who had not Asperger's disorder, but possibly other disorders. The combination of the subscale scores and the Asperger's Disorder Quotient distinguished between these two groups with an accuracy rate of 83%. The subscale scores and the Asperger's Disorder Quotient were significantly higher in a group of individuals diagnosed with Asperger's disorder than individuals diagnosed with autistic disorder, individuals with other disabilities, and individuals without disabilities.

Norms The GADS was standardized on 371 individuals aged 3–22 years who had been diagnosed with Asperger's disorder. Raw scores were converted to standard scores and percentiles.

Use A manual and rating scales enabling direct scoring are available from the publisher at the address below.

Key references

Gilliam JE. GADS: Gilliam Asperger's Disorder Scale. Examiner's Manual. Austin: PRO-ED, Inc, 2001.

Address

PRO-ED, Inc.
8700 Shoal Creek Boulevard
Austin, Texas 78757–6897
USA
www.proedinc.com

Gilliam Asperger's Disorder Scale – sample items

		Never observed	Seldom observed	Sometimes observed	Frequently observed
3.	Has difficulty playing with other children	0	1	2	3
9.	Expresses feelings of frustration and anger inappropriately	0	1	2	3
12.	Is unaware or insensitive to the needs of others	0	1	2	3
17.	Displays clumsy and uncoordinated gross motor movements	0	1	2	3
22.	Attaches very concrete meanings to words	0	1	2	3
27.	Has difficulty identifying when someone is teasing	0	1	2	3

Note. From Summary/Response Booklet, Gilliam Asperger's Disorder Scale, by James E Gilliam, 2001, Austin, TX: PRO-ED. www.proedinc.com. Copyright 2001 by PRO-ED, Inc. Reprinted with permission.

Gilliam Autism Rating Scale-Second Edition (GARS-2)

Time 10 minutes

Ages 3–22

Time Frame Not specified.

Purpose Assessment of autistic behaviors.

Commentary

The GARS-2 is based on the definition of autism adopted by the Autism Society of America and on diagnostic criteria for autistic disorder in the DSM-IV.

Versions

The Gilliam Autism Rating Scale-Second Edition (GARS-2) consists of one form that can be completed by parents and professionals at home and school.

Properties

Items The GARS-2 comprises 42 items assessing observed behaviors that are rated on a 4-point scale with responses: never observed, seldom observed, sometimes observed, and frequently observed. In addition, the GARS-2 comprises 20 items about a child's development before age 3 years that are rated on a 2-point scale with responses: yes, and no. The GARS-2 also comprises several open-ended questions to help examiners reach a conclusion.

Scales The items about observed behaviors of the GARS-2 are scored on three subscales which are labeled: Stereotyped behaviors, Communication, and Social Interaction. In addition, the Autism Index is computed by summing subscales and converting the sum into a quotient. The yes-no items are not scored on subscales.

Reliability Test–retest correlations across a 1-week interval ranged from 0.70 to 0.90 for the subscales and the correlation was 0.88 for the Autism Index in a sample of children with autism.

Cronbach's alphas ranged from 0.84 to 0.88 for the subscales and 0.94 for the Autism Index in the normative sample.

Validity Correlations between the GARS-2 subscales and corresponding subscales of a parent-reported measure of autistic behavior ranged from 0.56 to 0.78, while correlations between non-corresponding subscales ranged from 0.22 to 0.65. Total scores of both measures correlated 0.64.

Subscale scores and the Autism Index were significantly higher in a groups of individuals diagnosed with autistic disorder than groups of individuals who had intellectual disabilities, had multiple disabilities, or had no disabilities. The Autism Index distinguished individuals diagnosed with autism from individuals who had intellectual disabilities with a sensitivity of 85% and a specificity of 85%, from individuals who had multiple disabilities with a sensitivity of 84% and a specificity of 84%, and from individuals who had no disabilities with a sensitivity of 100% and a specificity of 87%.

Norms The GARS-2 was standardized on 1107 individuals aged 3–22 years who had been diagnosed as autistic. Raw scores were converted to standard scores and percentiles.

Use A manual and rating scales enabling direct scoring are available from the publisher at the address below.

Key references

Gilliam JE. GARS-2: Gilliam Autism Rating Scale-Second Edition. Examiner's Manual. Austin: PRO-ED, Inc, 2005.

Address

PRO-ED, Inc.
8700 Shoal Creek Boulevard
Austin, Texas 78757–6897
USA
www.proedinc.com

Gilliam Autism Rating Scale – Second Edition (GARS-2) – sample items

		Never observed	Seldom observed	Sometimes observed	Frequently observed
9.	Rocks back and forth while seated or standing	0	1	2	3
12.	Flaps hands or fingers in front of face or at sides	0	1	2	3
17.	Repeats words or phrases over and over	0	1	2	3
27.	Uses gestures instead of speech or signs to obtain objects	0	1	2	3
33.	Withdraws, remains aloof, or acts standoffish in group situations	0	1	2	3
40.	Becomes upset when routines are changed	0	1	2	3

Note. From Summary/Response Booklet, Gilliam Autism Rating Scale-Second Edition, by James E Gilliam, 2006, Austin, TX: PRO-ED. www.proedinc.com Copyright 2006 by PRO-ED, Inc. Reprinted with permission.

Infant Behavioral Summarized Evaluation (IBSE)

Time 10–15 minutes

Ages 1/2–4

Time Frame Not specified.

Purpose Assessment of autistic behaviors.

Commentary

The IBSE is adapted from the Behavioral Summarized Evaluation (BSE; Barthélémy et al, 1990) and is specifically designed to assess autistic behavior of young children.

Versions

The Infant Behavioral Summarized Evaluation (IBSE) is intended to be completed by clinicians who have observed children.

Properties

Items The IBSE comprises 33 items which are rated on a 5-point scale with responses: never observed, sometimes, often, very often, and continuously.

Scales Factor analysis was used to determine the structure of the IBSE. Two factors were identified: a factor labeled Autism, and a second factor which comprises only three items.

Reliability Kappas of ratings between two raters as a measure of interrater reliability were above 0.40 for 31 items and below 0.40 for two items. The intraclass reliability of the total score based on the 33 items was 0.97.

Validity All 19 item ratings of the Autism factor were significantly higher for children diagnosed with autism than for children diagnosed with mental retardation and than children with no diagnoses. Discriminant analysis indicated that the 19 items of the Autism factor correctly classified 83% of the children diagnosed with autism and children diagnosed with mental retardation with a sensitivity of 85% and specificity of 82%. The 19 items of the Autism correctly classified 95% of the children diagnosed with autism and children with no diagnoses with a sensitivity of 92% and specificity of 100%

Norms No information reported.

Use The scale can be found in Adrien et al. (1992).

Key references

Adrien JL, Barthélémy C, Perrot A, et al. Validity and reliability of the Infant Behavioral Summarized Evaluation (IBSE): A rating scale for the assessment of young children with autism and developmental disorders. J Autism Dev Disord 1992; 22: 375–94.

Barthélémy C, Adrien JL, Tanguay P, et al. The Behavior Summarized Evaluation: Validity and reliability of a scale for the assessment of autistic behaviors. J Autism Dev Disord 1990; 20: 189–204.

Address

Jean-Louis Adrien
UFR de Psychologie
Université René Descartes – Paris 5
71, av. Edouard Vaillant
92100 Boulogne-Billancourt
Paris
France
Jean-louis.adrien@univ-paris5.fr

Krug Asperger's Disorder Index (KADI)

Time 5 minutes

Ages 6–21

Time Frame Not specified

Purpose Assessment of Asperger's disorder behavior.

Commentary

The KADI was developed to serve three goals: 1) to identify individuals who have Asperger's disorder, 2) to target goals for intervention, and 3) to be used in research on Asperger's disorder.

Versions

The Krug Asperger's Disorder Index (KADI) consists of one form that can be completed by parents and professionals at home and school.

Properties

Items   The KADI comprises 32 items which are rated on weighted item responses. Each item has its own fixed response. Responses range from 0 to 4.

Scales   The items are scored on one total score which is a weighted sum of the ratings.

Reliability   Test–retest correlation across a 2-week interval was 0.98 in a sample of individuals with Asperger's disorder.

   Cronbach's alpha was 0.93 and the split-half reliability was 0.89 in a sample of individuals with Asperger's disorder.

Validity   The total score was significantly higher in a group of individuals diagnosed with Asperger's disorder than a group of individuals diagnosed with autistic disorder. The total score of the KADI distinguished between individuals diagnosed with Asperger's disorder

and those without that disorder with a sensitivity of 78% and a specificity of 94%.

Norms   The KADI was standardized on samples of individuals aged 6–21 years: 130 diagnosed with Asperger's disorder, 162 diagnosed with autistic disorder, and 194 from the general population. Raw scores were converted to standard scores and percentiles.

Use   A manual and rating scales enabling direct scoring are available from the publisher at the address below.

Key references

Krug DA, Arick JR. KADI: Krug Asperger's Disorder Index. Examiner's Manual. Austin: PRO-ED, Inc, 2003.

Address

PRO-ED, Inc.
8700 Shoal Creek Boulevard
Austin, Texas 78757–6897
USA
www.proedinc.com

Krug Asperger's Disorder Index (KADI) – sample items

	Elementary: ages 6–11	
	Column A	Column B
2. Conversationally, talks about single subject excessively	3	4
7. Says things that may embarrass others	3	3
17. Has very high standards for self and others		4
23. Not dependent on others for their help and advice		3
30. Seems possible might someday live by self, independently		4

Note. From Profile/Examiner Record Form, Krug Asperger's Disorder Index, by David A Krug and Joel R Arick, 2003, Austin, TX: PRO-ED. www.proedinc.com Copyright 2003 by PRO-ED, Inc. Reprinted with permission.

Modified Checklist for Autism in Toddlers (M-CHAT)

Time 5 minutes

Ages 18–30 months

Time Frame Not specified

Purpose Assessment of autistic behaviors.

Commentary

The M-CHAT is a modification of the Checklist for Autism in Toddlers (CHAT; Baron-Cohen et al., 1992). It includes the 9 parent-report items from the CHAT and additional items pertaining to symptoms in very young children.

Versions

The Modified Checklist for Autism in Toddlers (M-CHAT) is a parent report only.

Properties

Items   The M-CHAT comprises 23 items that are rated on a 2-point scale with responses: yes, and no.

Scales   The items are scored on a total score. In addition, 6 items found to be the best discriminators of children with autism spectrum disorders can be scored on a separate scale.

Reliability   Cronbach's alpha was 0.85 for the total score and 0.83 for the 6-item scale.

Validity   Both the total score and the 6-item score were significantly higher in a group of children with autism spectrum disorder than in groups of children without autism spectrum disorder. Various cut-off values identified children with autism spectrum disorder with sensitivities ranging from 87% to 97% and specificities ranging from 95% to 99%.

Norms   No information available.

Use   The M-CHAT is printed in Robins et al. (2001).

Key references

Baron-Cohen S, Allen J, Gillberg C. Can autism be detected at 18 months? The needle, the haystack, and the CHAT. Br J Psychiatry 1992; 161: 839–43.

Robins DL, Fein D, Barton ML, Green JA. The Modified Checklist for Autism in Toddlers: An initial study investigating the early detection of autism and pervasive developmental disorders. J Autism Dev Disord 2001; 31: 131–44.

Address

Diana L. Robins
Department of Psychology
University of Connecticut
406 Babbidge Road, U-1029
Storrs, Connecticut 06269–1020
USA

Modified Checklist for Autism in Toddlers (M-CHAT)

Please fill out the following about how your child **usually** is. Please try to answer every question. If the behavior is rare (e.g., you've seen it once or twice), please answer as if the child does not do it.

1.	Does your child enjoy being swung, bounced on your knee, etc?	Yes	No
2.	Does your child take an interest in other children?	Yes	No
3.	Does your child like climbing on things, such as up stairs?	Yes	No
4.	Does you child enjoy playing peek-a-boo/hide-and-seek?	Yes	No
5.	Does your child ever pretend, for example, to talk on the phone or take care of dolls, or pretend other things?	Yes	No
6.	Does your child ever use his/her index finger to point, to ask for something?	Yes	No
7.	Does your child ever use his/her index finger to point, to indicate interest in something?	Yes	No
8.	Can your child play properly with small toys (e.g. cars or bricks) without just mouthing, fiddling, or dropping them?	Yes	No
9.	Does your child ever bring objects over to you (parent) to show you something?	Yes	No
10.	Does your child look you in the eye for more than a second or two?	Yes	No
11.	Does your child ever seem oversensitive to noise? (e.g. plugging ears)	Yes	No
12.	Does your child smile in response to your face or your smile?	Yes	No
13.	Does your child imitate you? (e.g., you make a face – will your child imitate it?)	Yes	No
14.	Does your child respond to his/her name when you call?	Yes	No
15.	If you point at a toy across the room, does your child look at it?	Yes	No
16.	Does your child walk?	Yes	No
17.	Does your child look at things you are looking at?	Yes	No
18.	Does your child make unusual finger movements near his/her face?	Yes	No
19.	Does your child try to attract your attention to his/her own activity?	Yes	No
20.	Have you ever wondered if your child is deaf?	Yes	No
21.	Does your child understand what people say?	Yes	No
22.	Does your child sometimes stare at nothing or wander with no purpose?	Yes	No
23.	Does your child look at your face to check your reaction when faced with something unfamiliar?	Yes	No

Reproduced from Robins DL et al. J Autism Dev Disorders 2001; 31:131–44 with kind permission of Springer Science and Business media.

PDD Behavior Inventory (PDDBI)

Time Standard versions: 20–30 minutes; Extended versions: 30–45 minutes

Ages 11/2–121/2

Time Frame Not specified

Purpose Assessment of problem behaviors and social communication skills.

Commentary

The PDDBI was developed to provide an assessment scale of adaptive, as well as maladaptive behaviors, that could be used to evaluate change of functioning, and would be useful for multiple applications, such as clinical, medical, educational, and research.

Versions

The PDD Behavior Inventory (PDDBI) comprises a parent-report (PDDBI-P) and a teacher-report (PDDBI-T) form. Both forms are available in two versions: a standard and an extended (PDDBI-PX and PDDBI-TX) version which comprises a half more items than the standard version.

Properties

Items   The four versions of the PDDBI comprise different numbers of items: The PDDBI-P comprises 124 items, the PDDBI-T 124 items, the PDDBI-PX 188 items, and the PDDBI-TX 180 items. All items are rated on a 5-point scale with responses: does not show the behavior, rarely shows the behavior, sometimes/partially shows the behavior, usually/typically shows the behavior, and don't understand. An examiner can go over items for which a respondent gave a don't understand response.

Scales   Principal component analysis and internal consistency analyses were used to select and evaluate items and to form scales. The items of the PDDBI are grouped into clusters, most containing four items. Each cluster addresses a specific behavior, for example the cluster Visual Behaviors comprises four items which all pertain to staring or looking. There are 29–44 clusters, depending on the version of the PDDBI. Cluster scores are the simple sums of the four items of each cluster.

The clusters are grouped into domains. For example, the Ritualisms/Resistance to Change domain comprises the Resistance to Change in the Environment, Resistance to change in Schedules/Routines, and Rituals clusters. The extended versions comprise 10 domains and the standard versions comprise 6 domains from the extended versions that are most pertinent to the diagnosis of autism. The domains are labeled: Sensory/Perceptual Approach Behaviors; Ritualisms/Resistance to Change; Social Pragmatic Problems; Semantic/Pragmatic Problems; Arousal Regulation Problems; Specific Fears; Aggressiveness; Social Approach Behaviors; Expressive Language; and Learning, Memory, and Receptive Language. The domains can be classified into two sections: Approach/Withdrawal Problems, and Receptive/Expressive Social Communication Abilities.

In addition, composite scores can be formed by summing domain scores. The composite scores are labeled: Repetitive, Ritualistic, and Pragmatic Problems; Approach/Withdrawal Problems; Expressive Social Communication Abilities; Receptive/Expressive Social Communication Abilities; and Autism. The domains constituting the Autism composite score were selected because of their resemblance with DSM-IV criteria for autism and associated non-diagnostic behaviors.

Reliability   Test–retest correlations ranged from 0.60 to 0.90 across a 2-week interval for the teacher-reported domain and composite scores, 0.58–0.99 across a 6-month interval for parent-reported and teacher-reported domain and composite scores, and 0.38–0.91 across a 12-month interval for parent-reported domain and composite scores.

Cronbach's alphas ranged from 0.83 to 0.98 for the parent-reported and from 0.81 to 0.98 for the teacher reported domain and composite scores.

Validity   The Autism composite score correlated 0.48 for the parent form and 0.32 for the teacher form with a clinician-reported measure of autism severity. The correlations of autism severity with Receptive/Expressive Social Communication Abilities scores were generally higher than the correlations with Approach/Withdrawal Problems scores. The parent-reported and teacher-reported PDDBI scales correlated moderately with corresponding scales of different parent-reported and teacher-reported measures of problem behavior, socialization and communication skills.

The Autism composite score differed significantly among children classified into three groups consisting of children diagnosed with autism, diagnosed within the autism spectrum, and with no autism according to a diagnostic interview with parents and observational assessment. Most other scales and composite scores of the PDDBI differed significantly among the three groups as well.

Norms   The PDDBI was standardized on ratings by 369 parents and 277 teachers of clinical children ranging in age from 1 year 6 months to 12 years 5 months. Raw scores are converted to age-adjusted T-scores for the domain and composite scores and are converted to percentile ranges for the cluster scores.

Use   A manual, rating forms, score summary sheets, profile forms, and a scoring program are available from the publisher at the address below.

Key references

Cohen IL. Criterion-related validity of the PDD Behavior Inventory. J Autism Dev Disord 2003; 33: 47–53.

Cohen IL, Sudhalter V. PDDBI – PDD Behavior Inventory: Professional Manual. Lutz, FL: Psychological Assessment Resources, Inc, 2005.

Cohen IL. The PDD Behavior Inventory: A rating scale for assessing response to intervention in children with pervasive developmental disorder. J Autism Dev Disord 2003; 33: 31–45.

Address

Psychological Assessment Resources, Inc.
16204 N. Florida Avenue
Lutz, FL 33549
USA
www.parinc.com

PDD Behavior Inventory (PDDBI) – sample items – Parent Rating Form

	Does not show behavior	Rarely shows behavior	Sometimes/partially shows behavior	Usually/typically shows behavior	Don't understand
26. Resists changing from one activity to another when requested to do so by familiar people	0	1	2	3	?
114. Smiles when a familiar song is sung, when a familiar name is mentioned, when he/she sees a familiar picture, etc.	0	1	2	3	?

Pervasive Developmental Disorders Screening Test-II (PDDST-II)

Time 15 minutes

Ages 1 1/2–8

Time Frame Each item addresses one out of the following age ranges: birth to 6 months, 6 to 12 months, 12 to 18 months, 18 to 24 months, 24 to 30 months, and 30 to 36 months.

Purpose Assessment of autistic behaviors.

Commentary

The PDDST-II was designed for early identification of autism spectrum disorders. It comprises items specific to development in the first 48 months of life.

Versions

The Pervasive Developmental Disorders Screening Test-II (PDDST-II) is a parent report that comes in three versions indicating three stages of screening in different clinical settings: Stage 1–Primary Care Screener (Stage 1–PCS), Stage 2–Developmental Clinic Screener (Stage 2–DCS), and Stage 3–Autism Clinic Severity Screener (Stage 3–ACSS).

Properties

Items The PDDST-II contains items specific for each form and items common on all forms. The Stage 1–PCS comprises 22 items, the Stage 2–DCS 14 items, and the Stage 3–ACSS 12 items. In addition to these screening items, the manual provides 41 supplemental items for obtaining more information about children's behaviors from parents. Screening and supplemental items are rated on a 2-point scale with responses: yes, usually true; and no, usually not true.

Scales The items of each form are scored on a total score which is the count of the yes responses.

Reliability No information provided.

Validity Sensitivities and specificities of the PDDST-II for distinguishing children diagnosed with and without autism spectrum disorder in the standardization sample were 92% and 91%, respectively for the Stage 1–PCS, 73% and 49%, respectively for the Stage 2–DCS, and 58% and 60%, respectively for the Stage 3–ACSS.

Norms The PDDST-II was standardized on 687 children referred for autism spectrum disorder to an autism clinic and 256 children with a very low birth weight who were used as a comparison group. Cut-off scores are used for identifying children with autism spectrum disorder.

Use A manual and rating scales can be obtained from the publisher at the address below.

Key references

Siegel B. PDDST-II Pervasive Developmental Disorders Screening Test-II. San Antonio: The Psychological Corporation, 2004.

Address

Harcourt Assessment
Procter House
1 Procter Street
London WC1V 6EU
United Kingdom
www.harcourt-uk.com

Real Life Rating Scale (RLRS)

Time 10–15 minutes

Ages 6–16

Time Frame Ratings are based on 30–minutes observation periods.

Purpose Assessment of autistic behaviors.

Commentary

The RLRS was designed to assess autistic behaviors of patients in their natural settings without modifications or experimental constraints. It was specifically designed for assessing short-term responses to treatments and to be completed by rapidly trained non-professional observers.

Versions

The Real Life Rating Scale (RLRS) is intended to be completed by trained non-professional raters who observed children in real life settings.

Properties

Items   The RLRS comprises 47 items which are rated on a 4-point scale with responses: never, rarely, frequently, and almost always.

Scales   The items of the RLRS are scored on five subscales which are labeled: Sensory-motor, Social-relationship to people, Affectual response, Sensory response, and Language.

Reliability   Median interrater correlations for the 47 items was 0.44 among inexperienced raters and 0.70 among experienced raters.

Validity   The subscales of the RLRS correlated significantly with clinician-reported autistic behaviors, except for the Sensory-motor scale which has no counterpart in the other measure.

Norms   No information reported.

Use   The rating scale, its scoring instructions and behavior descriptions are given in Freeman et al. (1986).

Key references

Freeman BJ, Ritvo ER, Yokota A, Ritvo A. A scale for rating symptoms of patients with the syndrome of autism in real life settings. J Am Acad Child Adolesc Psychiatry 1986; 25: 130–6.

Address

B. J. Freeman
Neuropsychiatric Institute
760 Westwood Plaza
Los Angeles, CA 90024
USA

Real Life Rating Scale (RLRS)

Subject's name _____   ID: _____

Description and time of setting: _____   Visit: _____

People present: _____   Date: _____

Never = 0; rarely = 1; frequently = 2; almost always = 3

Scale I

Sensory motor behaviors

1. Whirls _____
2. Flaps _____
3. Pacing _____
4. Bangs/hits self _____
5. Rocks _____
6. Toe walks _____
7. Other _____

Sum I: _____

Mean: _____

Scale II

Social relationship to people

*1. Appropriate response to interaction attempt _____
*2. Appropriate response to activities in environment _____
*3. Initiates appropriate physical interaction _____
4. Ignores interaction attempt _____
5. Disturbs others _____
6. Changes activities _____
7. Genital manipulation _____
8. Isolates self _____
9. Response to hug/being held by rigidity _____

Sum II: _____

Mean: _____

Scale III

Affectual reactions

1. Abrupt change _____
2. Grimaces _____
3. Temper outbursts/unpredictability _____
4. Cries _____
5. Other _____

Sum III: _____

Mean: _____

Scale IV

Sensory responses

*1. Uses objects appropriately _____
2. Agitated by noises _____
3. Whirls/spins objects _____
4. Rubs surfaces _____
5. Agitated by new activity _____
6. Watches motion hand/object _____
7. Repetitive/stereotypic _____
8. Sniffs self or objects _____
9. Lines up objects _____
10. Visual detail/scrutiny _____
11. Destructive to objects _____
12. Repetitive vocalizations _____
13. Stares _____
14. Covers ears or eyes _____
15. Flicks _____
16. Other _____

Sum IV: _____

Mean: _____

Scale V

Language

*1. Communicative use of language _____
*2. Initiates or responds to communication _____
*3. Initiates appropriate verbal communication _____
4. Noncommunicative use of D. Echolalia _____
5. Immediate echolalia _____
6. Delusions _____
7. Auditory hallucination _____
8. Visual hallucination _____
9. Noncommunicative vocalizations _____
10. No or brief response to communication attempts _____

Sum V: _____

Mean: _____

Overall scale

Sum:

I _____   II _____   III _____   IV _____   V _____   ÷ 5 = _____

*Score or behavior is subtracted from others before computing the mean.

Social Communication Questionnaire (SCQ)

Time 10 minutes

Ages 4–40

Time Frame Lifetime: entire life

Current: last 3 months

Purpose Assessment of autistic behaviors.

Commentary

The SCQ was designed as companion screening instrument for the Autism Diagnostic Interview-Revised (ADI-R; Rutter et al, 2003b). Items were selected to match the content of the ADI-R, but the SCQ is briefer.

Versions

The Social Communication Questionnaire (SCQ) is available as a parent report and comes in two versions: Lifetime and Current.

Properties

Items   The SCQ comprises 40 items that are rated on a 2-point scale with responses: yes, and no.

Scales   The items can be scored on the total score which is the simple sum of all item ratings. In addition, the items can be scored on subscales that correspond to domains on the ADI-R, although these domains were not in agreement with factor analysis of the SCQ. The subscales are: Reciprocal Social Interaction; Communication; and Restricted, Repetitive, and Stereotyped Patterns.

Reliability   Cronbach's alpha for the total score was 0.90 in the standardization sample. Cronbach's alphas for the total score ranged from 0.84 to 0.93 across age groups and from 0.81 to 0.92 across diagnostic groups in a screening sample.

Validity   Total scores of the SCQ and the ADI-R correlated 0.71, and correlations between corresponding subscales of the SCQ and ADI-R ranged from 0.55 to 0.89.

Individuals with autistic disorder or autism spectrum disorder had significantly higher subscale and total scores than individuals without these disorders. Individuals with autistic disorder had significantly higher subscale and total scores than individuals with other autism spectrum disorders. The total score distinguished autism spectrum disorder from other disorders with a sensitivity of 85% and a specificity of 75%.

Norms   The SCQ was standardized on 200 ratings of individuals aged 4–40 years who participated in clinical studies.

Use   A manual and rating scale enabling direct scoring are available from the publisher at the address below.

Key references

Berument SK, Rutter M, Lord C, Pickles A, Bailey A. Autism screening questionnaire: diagnostic validity. Br J Psychiatry 1999; 175: 444–51.

Rutter M, Bailey A, Lord C. The Social Communication Questionnaire Manual. Los Angeles: Western Psychological Services, 2003a.

Rutter M, Le Couteur A, Lord C. Autism Diagnostic Interview-Revised Manual. Los Angeles: Western Psychological Services, 2003b.

Address

Western Psychological Services
12031 Wilshire Blvd.
Los Angeles, CA 90025–1251
USA
www.wpspublish.com

Social Communication Questionnaire (SCQ) – sample items

5.	Does she/he ever get her/his pronouns mixed up (e.g., saying *you* or *she/he* for *I*)?	yes	no
8.	Does she/he ever have things that she/he seems to have to do in a very particular way or order or rituals that she/he insists that you go through?	yes	no
15.	Does she/he ever have any mannerisms or odd ways of moving her/his hands or fingers, such as flapping or moving her/his fingers in front of her/his eyes?	yes	no
19.	Does she/he have any particular friends or a best friend?	yes	no
21.	Does she/he ever *spontaneously* copy you (or other people) or what you are doing (such as vacuuming, gardening, or mending things)?	yes	no
33.	Does she/he show a normal range of facial expressions?	yes	no

Social Responsiveness Scale (SRS)

Time 15 minutes

Age 4–18

Time Frame Last 6 months

Purpose Assessment of autistic behaviors.

Commentary

The SRS is a screening and diagnostic instrument for assessing autism spectrum conditions. It does not present autism as a disorder that is present or absent, but as a quantitative scale as is suggested by research in the past 10 years indicating autism conceptualized as a spectrum condition.

Versions

The Social Responsiveness Scale (SRS) consists of one form that can be completed by parents or teachers.

Properties

Items   The SRS comprises 65 items that are rated on a 4-point scale with responses: not true, sometimes true, often true, and almost always true.

Scales   The items are scored on a total score by summing all item ratings. The items can also be scored on 5 treatment subscales which are labeled: Social Awareness, Social Cognition, Social Communication, Social Motivation, and Autistic Mannerisms. These scales are based on expert judgements of the SRS items. The treatment scales are not used for screening or diagnosis, but are useful in designing and evaluating treatment programs. Factor analysis could not support the composition of subscales, but suggested a single, continuously distributed factor.

Reliability   Test–retest correlations for the total score across a 17-month interval were 0.85 for males and 0.77 for females in a sample of 379 individuals who took part in a twin study.

Cronbach's alphas for the total score ranged from 0.93 to 0.97 in normative and clinical samples. Cronbach's alphas for the subscales ranged from 0.77 to 0.90 in a clinical sample.

Validity   Children with PDD-NOS had significantly higher total scores than children with conduct disorder, psychotic disorder, mood disorder, and ADHD.

Using a parent interview for establishing a clinical diagnosis of autism, child psychiatric patients were classified into three groups: children with autism, children with Asperger's disorder or PDD-NOS, and children with non-PDD disorders. The total scores of the first two groups were significantly higher than of the third group. Furthermore, correlations between mother, father, and teacher total scores of the SRS and the scores obtained with the diagnostic parent interview were significant and ranged from 0.52 to 0.79.

Cut-off values for the total score of the SRS identify any autism spectrum disorder with a sensitivity of 0.77 and a specificity of 0.75.

Norms   The SRS was standardized on 1636 ratings obtained from several samples including children age 4–18 years. Raw scores were converted to T-scores.

Use   A manual, rating scales enabling direct scoring or enabling computerized scoring are available from the publisher at the address below.

Key references

Constantino JN, Gruber CP. Social Responsiveness Scale (SRS). Manual. Los Angeles: Western Psychological Services, 2005.

Constantino JN, Przybeck T, Friesen D, Todd RD. Reciprocal social behavior in children with and without pervasive developmental disorders. J Dev Behav Pediatr 2000; 21: 2–11.

Address

Western Psychological Services
12031 Wilshire Blvd.
Los Angeles, CA 90025–1251
USA
www.wpspublish.com

Social Responsiveness Scale (SRS) – sample items

1 = NOT TRUE 2 = SOMETIMES TRUE 3 = OFTEN TRUE 4 = ALMOST TRUE

2.	Expressions on his or her face don't match what he or she is saying.	1	2	3	4
5.	Doesn't recognize when others are trying to take advantage of him or her.	1	2	3	4
6.	Would rather be alone than with others.	1	2	3	4
14.	Is not well coordinated.	1	2	3	4
24.	Has more difficulty making friends, even when trying his or her best.	1	2	3	4
32.	Has good personal hygiene.	1	2	3	4
40.	Is imaginative, good at pretending (without losing touch with reality).	1	2	3	4
43.	Separates easily from caregivers.	1	2	3	4
50.	Has repetitive, odd behaviors such as hand flapping or rocking.	1	2	3	4
57.	Gets teased a lot.	1	2	3	4

3.8 ADHD

ADHD Rating Scale-IV (ADHD RS-IV)

Time 5 minutes

Ages 4–20

Time Frame Last 6 months

Purpose Assessment of ADHD problems.

Commentary

The first edition of the ADHD Rating Scale appeared in 1991 (DuPaul, 1991) and was based on the DSM-III-R criteria for ADHD. The ADHD Rating Scale-IV was revised to make the items compatible with the DSM-IV criteria for ADHD. In addition, the response scale was modified to reflect frequency of behavior.

Versions

The ADHD Rating Scale-IV (ADHD RS-IV) is available in two versions. The ADHD Rating Scale-IV: Home Version is to be completed by parents and the ADHD Rating Scale-IV: School Version is to be completed by teachers.

Properties

Items The ADHD Rating Scale-IV comprises 18 items that are rated on a 4-point scale with responses: never or rarely, sometimes, often, very often.

Scales The items are scored on two subscales which are supported by factor analysis. The subscales are: Inattention, and Hyperactivity-Impulsivity. In addition, the Total score is the sum of all item ratings.

Reliability Test–retest correlations for Inattention, Hyperactivity-Impulsivity, and the Total score across a 4-week interval were 0.78, 0.86, and 0.85, respectively for the ADHD Rating Scale-IV: Home Version, and 0.89, 0.88, and 0.90, respectively for the ADHD Rating Scale-IV: School Version in a sample of school children.

Cronbach's alphas for Inattention, Hyperactivity-Impulsivity, and the Total score were 0.86, 0.88, and 0.92, respectively for the ADHD Rating Scale-IV: Home Version, and 0.96, 0.88, and 0.94, respectively for the

ADHD Rating Scale-IV: School Version in a sample of school children.

Validity Subscales of the Rating Scale-IV: Home Version correlated significantly with parent-reported impulsivity and hyperactivity, conduct problems, and learning problems: 0.45, 0.45, and 0.66, respectively for Inattention, and 0.78, 0.65, and 0.45, respectively for Hyperactivity-Impulsivity. The subscales correlated also significantly with teacher-reported hyperactivity, and conduct problems: 0.38 and 0.39, respectively for Inattention, and 0.35 and 0.26, respectively for Hyperactivity-Impulsivity. Inattention only correlated significantly with teacher-reported attention problems (0.32). Neither subscale correlated significantly with parent-reported and teacher-reported anxiety. Of the correlations between the subscales and classroom observations of off-task behavior, fidgets, and accuracy, only the correlation between Inattention and accuracy was significant (–0.43).

Subscales of the Rating Scale-IV: School Version correlated significantly with teacher-reported attention problems, hyperactivity, conduct problems, and anxiety: 0.85, 0.73, 0.29, and 0.47, respectively for Inattention, and 0.44, 0.79, 0.55, and 0.25, respectively for Hyperactivity-Impulsivity. Correlations between the subscales and classroom observations of off-task behavior, fidgets, and accuracy were significant for Inattention (0.35, 0.28, –0.46, respectively), but for Hyperactivity-Impulsivity only the correlation with accuracy was significant (–0.34).

Among three groups of clinical children classified as having ADHD inattentive subtype (ADHD/I), ADHD combined subtype (ADHD/COM), and no ADHD (control group) parent and teacher Inattention scores were significantly higher for the ADHD/I and ADHD/COM groups than the control group, parent and teacher Hyperactivity-Impulsivity scores for the ADHD/COM groups were significantly higher than both other groups.

Norms The ADHD Rating Scale-IV was standardized on 2000 parent ratings and 2000 teacher ratings of school children aged 4–20 years representative of the US general population.

Use A manual which contains both rating scales in English and the Home Version in Spanish and scoring sheets is available from the publisher at the address below.

Key references

DuPaul GJ. Parent teacher ratings of ADHD symptoms: Psychometric properties in a community-based sample. J Clin Child Psychol 1991; 20: 245–53.

DuPaul GJ, Power TJ, Anastopoulos AD, Reid R. ADHD Rating Scale-IV Checklists, Norms, and Clinical Interpretation. New York, The Guilford Press, 1998.

Address

The Guilford Press
72 Spring Street
New York, NY 10012
USA
www.guilford.com

ADHD Symptoms Rating Scale (ADHD-SRS)

Time 10–15 minutes

Ages 5–18

Time Frame Last 3 months

Purpose Assessment of ADHD problems.

Commentary

The ADHD-SRS was designed to assess ADHD symptoms which are summarized in two subscales based on the two DSM-IV categories of ADHD: hyperactivity-impulsivity and inattention.

Versions

The ADHD Symptoms Rating Scale (ADHD-SRS) is available as one form that can be completed by parents or teachers.

Properties

Items   The ADHD-SRS comprises 56 items that are rated on a 5-point scale with responses: behavior does not occur/no knowledge of behavior, behavior occurs one to several times a month, behavior occurs one to several times a week, behavior occurs one to several times a day, and behavior occurs one to several times an hour.

Scales   The items of the ADHD-SRS are scored on two subscales which were supported by factor analysis. The subscales are: Hyperactive-Impulsive, and Inattentive. In addition, a total score is computed by summing the subscale scores.

Reliability   Test–retest correlations across a 2-week interval ranged from 0.94 to 0.98 across age and scales of teacher ratings of elementary and middle school students.

Cronbach's alphas ranged from 0.92 to 0.99 across sex, age, scales, and informant in the standardization sample.

Validity   Correlations of the ADHD-SRS subscales and Total Score with corresponding scales of similar parent-

reported measurements were 0.90 and 0.92 for Inattentive, 0.90 and 0.94 for Hyperactive-Impulsive, and 0.91 and 0.94 for the total score. For teacher-reported measurements these correlations ranged from 0.76 to 0.93 for Inattentive, 0.93 to 0.95 for Hyperactive-Impulsive, and from 0.94 to 0.97 for the Total Score. Correlations of the teacher-reported ADHD-SRS subscales and the Total Score with teacher reported conduct problems ranged from 0.71 to 0.86, and with anxiety from 0.24 to 0.36.

Children diagnosed with ADHD had significantly higher scores on the subscales and the Total Score of both parent and teacher forms than children from the standardization sample who were matched on sex, age, and ethnicity.

Norms   The ADHD-SRS was standardized on 1341 parent ratings and 1486 teacher ratings of children aged 5–18 years from the US general population recruited through schools, individual educators, and psychologists. Raw scores are converted to T-scores and percentile ranks.

Use   A manual, rating scales enabling direct scoring, and a computer scoring program are available from the publisher at the address below.

Key references

Holland ML, Gimpel GA, Merrell KW. Innovations in assessing ADHD: Development, psychometric properties, and factor structure of the ADHD symptoms rating scale (ADHD-SRS). J Psychopathol Behav Assess 1998; 20: 307–32.

Holland ML, Gimpel GA, Merrell KW. ADHD-SRS ADHD Symptoms Rating Scale. Manual. Lutz, Fl: Psychological Assessment Resources, Inc, 2001.

Address

Psychological Assessment Resources, Inc.
16204 N. Florida Avenue
Lutz, FL 33549
USA
www.parinc.com

ADHD Symptoms Rating Scale (ADHD-SRS) – sample items

	Behavior does not occur/ No knowledge of behavior	Behavior occurs one to several times a month	Behavior occurs one to several times a week	Behavior occurs one to several times a day	Behavior occurs one to several times an hour
21. Shifts from one activity to another	0	1	2	3	4
47. Has difficulty concentrating	0	1	2	3	4

Attention Deficit Disorders Evaluation Scale – Third Edition (ADDES-3)

Time 20 minutes

Ages 4–18

Time Frame Not specified

Purpose Assessment of ADHD problems.

Commentary

The ADDES-3 was designed to assess ADHD characteristics based on the DSM-IV criteria for ADHD.

Versions

The Attention Deficit Disorders Evaluation Scale – Third Edition (ADDES-3) comprises two forms: the Attention Deficit Disorders Evaluation Scale – Third Edition Home Version (ADDES-3 HV) to be completed by parents or caregivers, and the Attention Deficit Disorders Evaluation Scale – Third Edition School Version (ADDES-3 SV) to be completed by teachers.

Properties

Items   The ADDES-3 HV comprises 46 items and the ADDES-3 SV 60 items. The items are rated on a 6-point scale with responses: not developmentally appropriate for age, not observed, one to several times per month, one to several times per week, one to several times per day, one to several times per hour.

Scales   Factor analysis supported the two theoretically derived subscales: Inattentive, and Hyperactive-Impulsive. The sum of the two subscales constitutes the Total Score.

Reliability   Test–retest correlations across a 30-day interval for Inattentive, Hyperactive-Impulsive, and Total Score are, respectively 0.86, 0.82, and 0.86 for the ADDES-3 HV, and, respectively 0.92, 0.88, and 0.91 for the ADDES-3 SV.

Cronbach's alphas for Inattentive, Hyperactive-Impulsive, and Total Score are, respectively 0.96, 0.96, and 0.98 for the ADDES-3 HV, and, respectively 0.98, 0.99, and 0.99 for the ADDES-3 SV.

Validity   The ADDES-3 HV subscale Inattentive correlated 0.76 and 0.83 with parent-reported measures of attention and Hyperactive-Impulsive correlated 0.78 and 0.88 with parent-reported measures of hyperactivity. Correlations between the ADDES-3 SV subscale Inattentive and teacher-reported measures of attention and hyperactivity ranged from 0.80 to 0.89, and correlations between Hyperactivity-Impulsive and teacher-reported measures of attention and hyperactivity ranged from 0.68 to 0.90.

Mean scores of both ADDES-3 SV subscales differed significantly between students identified with ADHD and students without ADHD.

Norms   The ADDES-3 HV was standardized on ratings of 2848 children and the ADDES-3 SV on ratings of 3903 children from the USA general population. Subscale raw scores were converted to standardized scores with mean 10 and standard deviation 3. The Total Score was converted to a standardized score with mean 100 and standard deviation 15 and into percentiles.

Use   Manuals, rating scales, an additional guide for parents, and an intervention manual are available from the publisher at the address below.

Key references

McGarney SB, Arthaud TJ. Attention Deficit Disorders Evaluation Scale - Third Edition. Columbia, Missouri: Hawthorne Educational Services, Inc, 2004.

Address

Hawthorne Educational Services, Inc.
800 Gray Oak Drive
Columbia, MO 65201
USA
www.hes-inc.com

Attention Deficit Disorders Evaluation Scale – Third Edition (ADDES-3) – sample items

Home Version

2. Does not listen to what others are saying
12. Has a short attention span (e.g., does not sit still while a story is being read, does not keep his/her attention on homework assignments, is easily distracted, etc.)
29. Begins things before receiving directions or instructions (e.g., putting things together, performing chores, using tools, etc.)
43. Runs in the house, does not sit appropriately on the furniture, yells, etc.

School Version

7. Needs oral questions and directions frequently repeated (e.g., student says, 'I don't understand,' needs constant reminders, etc.)
23. Does not remain on-task (e.g., is more interested in other activities, sits and does nothing, etc.)
34. Blurts out answers without being called on
58. Demonstrates inappropriate behavior when moving with a group (e.g., fails to stay in line, runs, pushes, etc.)

Attention-Deficit/Hyperactivity Disorder Test (ADHDT)

Time 5–10 minutes

Ages 3–23

Time Frame Not specified

Purpose Assessment of ADHD problems.

Commentary

The ADHDT was designed to identify individuals with ADHD based on DSM-IV criteria and problems reported in the professional literature.

Versions

The Attention-Deficit/Hyperactivity Disorder Test (ADHDT) is only available as one form that can be completed by parents, teachers, or other professionals.

Properties

Items The ADHDT comprises 36 items that are rated on a 3-point scale with responses: not a problem, mild problem, and severe problem.

Scales The items of the ADHDT are scored on 3 subscales: Hyperactivity, Impulsivity, and Inattention. A total score can be computed by summing all item scores. In addition, the ADHD Quotient can be computed by summing the subscale scores after converting them into standard scores.

Reliability Test–retest correlations for the subscales and the ADHD Quotient ranged from 0.85 to 0.94 across a 1-week interval among undergraduate students, and ranged from 0.85 to 0.92 among children of whom the majority was diagnosed with ADHD.

Cronbach's alphas for the subscales and the ADHD Quotient were all higher than 0.90 across gender, age, and informant among people with ADHD.

Validity Correlations between Hyperactivity and comparable scales of other teacher-reported measures ranged from 0.70 to 0.83, between Impulsivity and a comparable scale was 0.78, and between Inattention and comparable scales ranged from 0.78 to 0.95. Correlation between the ADHD Quotient and a comparable teacher-reported measure of ADHD was 0.88. Correlations of the subscales and the ADHD Quotient with teacher-reported conduct problems ranged from 0.13 to 0.80, and with teacher-reported anxiety ranged from 0.09 to 0.39.

Individuals diagnosed with ADHD had significantly higher scores on the subscales and the ADHD Quotient than those who were diagnosed with learning disability, emotional disturbance, intellectual disability, or who had no diagnosis. Only Impulsivity was not significantly different between those who were diagnosed with ADHD and those who were diagnosed with emotional disturbance. The ADHD Quotient distinguished between individuals diagnosed with ADHD and those without ADHD with a sensitivity of 88% and a specificity of 99%.

Norms The ADHDT was standardized on ratings by parents, teachers, and other professionals of 1279 individuals in the USA and Canada aged 3–23 years who had a diagnosis of ADHD. Raw scores were converted to standard scores and percentile ranks.

Use A manual and rating scales enabling direct scoring are available from the publisher at the address below.

Key references

Gilliam JE. Attention-Deficit/Hyperactivity Disorder Test: A Method for Identifying Individuals with ADHD. Examiner's Manual. Austin: PRO-ED, Inc, 1995.

Address

PRO-ED, Inc.
8700 Shoal Creek Boulevard
Austin, Texas 78757–6897
USA
www.proedinc.com

Attention-Deficit/Hyperactivity Disorder Test (ADHDT) – sample items

	Not a problem	Mild problem	Severe problem
3. Excessive running, jumping, climbing	0	1	2
8. Difficulty remaining seated	0	1	2
14. Acts before thinking	0	1	2
20. Interrupts conversations	0	1	2
25. Fails to finish projects	0	1	2
32. Easily distracted	0	1	2

Note. From Summary/Response Booklet, Attention-Deficit/Hyperactivity Disorder Test, by James E Gilliam, 1995, Austin, TX: PRO-ED. www.proedinc.com Copyright 1995 by PRO-ED, Inc. Reprinted with permission.

Brown Attention-Deficit Disorder Scales (Brown ADD Scales)

Time 10–20 minutes

Ages 3–18

Time Frame Last 6 months

Purpose Assessment of ADHD problems.

Commentary

The Brown ADD Scales are based on Thomas Brown's model of the ADD syndrome (Brown, 2005). The model's central theme is that children, adolescents, and adults with ADHD have executive function impairments encompassing several cognitive functions. Typical difficulties are: inattention difficulties, organizing work, sustaining effort for tasks, screening out distractions, keeping track of assignments and belongings, and excessive forgetfulness in daily activities. These difficulties are sometimes accompanied by impulsive or hyperactive behavior problems.

Versions

The Brown Attention-Deficit Disorder Scales (Brown ADD Scales) comprise parent-report and teacher-report forms for ages 3–7, parent-report, teacher-report, and self-report forms for ages 8–12, and self-report forms for ages 12–18. Self-report forms for ages 18 years and older also exist, but these will not be discussed here.

Properties

Items The various forms of the Brown ADD Scales comprise 40–50 items that are rated on a 4-point scale with responses: never, once a week or less, twice a week, and almost daily.

Scales The items of the Brown ADD Scales are grouped into 5 to 6 clusters. These clusters are: 1. Organizing, Prioritizing, and Activating to Work; 2. Focusing, Sustaining, and Shifting Attention to Tasks; 3. Regulating Alertness, Sustaining Effort, and Processing Speed; 4. Managing Frustration and Modulating Emotions; 5. Utilizing Working Memory and Accessing Recall; 6. Monitoring and Self-Regulating Action. Cluster 6 is only appropriate for ages 3–12. In addition, the sum

of clusters 1 to 5 constitutes the ADD-Inattention Total Score, and the sum of clusters 1 to 6 constitutes the ADD Combined Total Score.

Reliability Test–retest correlations of cluster and total scores for children aged 3–7 years across a 1–4-week interval ranged from 0.69 to 0.81 for parent ratings and 0.78 to 0.89 for teacher ratings. For children aged 8–12 these test-retest correlations ranged from 0.84 to 0.92 for parent ratings, 0.84 to 0.93 for teacher ratings, and from 0.45 to 0.69 for self ratings. The test-retest correlation of the total score for adolescents aged 12–18 years across a 2-week interval was 0.87 for self ratings.

Cronbach's alphas of cluster and total scores for children aged 3–7 years ranged from 0.73 to 0.97 for parent ratings and 0.80 to 0.98 for teacher ratings. Cronbach's alphas of cluster and total scores for children aged 8–12 years ranged from 0.74 to 0.98 for parent ratings, 0.76 to 0.98 for teacher ratings, and 0.71 to 0.96 for self ratings. Cronbach's alphas of cluster and total scores for adolescents aged 12–18 years ranged from 0.70 to 0.95 for self ratings.

Validity All clusters of the Brown ADD Scales correlated significantly with other parent- and teacher-reported measures of attention problems and hyperactivity. Cluster 4, which assesses problems in emotional regulation, correlated significantly with both internalizing and externalizing. Cluster 6 which assesses monitoring and self-regulating action correlated significantly with parent- and teacher-reported measures of impulsive or hyperactive behavior. Clusters 1, 2, 3, and 5 which assess executive functions correlated significantly with parent- and teacher-reported measures of cognitive problems.

Children and adolescents with high scores on the Brown ADD Scales are more impaired on IQ subtests that assess working memory and processing speed than other subtests.

Comparisons between groups of children diagnosed with ADHD and matched control groups of children not diagnosed with ADHD revealed that all cluster and total scores were significantly different in all age groups and for all informants.

Norms The Brown ADD Scales for children aged 3–12 years were standardized on a US population sample of 800 children and a clinical sample of 240 children. The

Brown ADD Scales for adolescents age 12–18 years were standardized on a US clinical sample of 190 adolescents diagnosed with ADHD and a matched control group of 190 students. Norm scores are presented as raw scores, T-scores, and cumulative percentage points.

Use   Further information about the Brown ADD Scales and Brown's model can be found on the website www.drthomasebrown.com. In addition to the rating scales, diagnostic forms are available which include a set of procedures for integrating a clinical history, a comorbidity screener, and a worksheet for integrating data from the Brown ADD Scales with standardized scores from other tests. Manuals, ratings scales which enable scoring, diagnostic forms, and software for scoring and reporting are available from the publisher at the address below.

Key references

Brown TE. Brown Attention-Deficit Disorder Scales. San Antonio, TX: The Psychological Corporation, 1996.

Brown TE. Brown Attention-Deficit Disorder Scales for Children and Adolescents. San Antonio, TX: The Psychological Corporation, 2001.

Brown TE. Attention Deficit Disorder: The unfocused mind in children and adults. New Haven, CT: Yale University Press, 2005.

Address

Harcourt Assessment
Procter House
1 Procter Street
London WC1V 6EV
UK
www.harcourt-uk.com

IOWA Conners Teacher's Rating Scale (IOWA Conners)

Time 5 minutes

Ages Grades K-6

Time Frame Not specified

Purpose Assessment of disruptive problems.

Commentary

The items of the IOWA Conners were a selection of 10 items from an early teacher version of the Conners' Rating Scales. Items pertaining to hyperactivity and aggression were selected to enable classification of children into four groups: children scoring high on both hyperactivity and aggression, children scoring high on hyperactivity and low on aggression, children scoring high on aggression and low on hyperactivity, and children scoring low on both hyperactivity and aggression.

Versions

The IOWA Conners Teacher Rating Scale (IOWA Conners) is available as a teacher report, but has also been used as a parent report and a self-report.

Properties

Items The IOWA Conners comprises 10 items that are rated on a 4-point scale with responses: not at all, just a little, pretty much, and very much.

Scales Factor analysis supported two subscales which are labeled: Inattentive/Overactive (I/O) and Oppositional/Defiant (O/D). In addition to the subscales, a total score can be computed as the sum of all items.

Reliability Test–retest correlations across a 1-week interval were 0.89 for the I/O subscale and 0.85 for the O/D subscale in elementary school children.

Cronbach's alphas were 0.87 and 0.89 for the I/O subscale and 0.82 and 0.85 for the O/D subscale in samples of elementary school children, and were 0.80 for the I/O subscale and 0.87 for the O/D subscale in clinical children.

Validity The IOWA Conners subscales correlated significantly with parent-reported and teacher-reported inattention, delinquency, and aggression.

Scores of the I/O and O/D subscales were significantly higher in clinical children than in elementary school children. The IOWA Conners was also sensitive to treatment.

Norms A table with means, standard deviations, and cut-off scores for 608 elementary school children in grades K-5 in the US can be found in Pelham (1989).

Use The IOWA Conners is printed in Loney and Milich (1982).

Key references

Casat CD, Norton HJ, Boyle-Whitesel M. Identification of elementary school children at risk for disruptive behavioral disturbance: Validation of a combined screening method. J Am Acad Child Adolesc Psychiatry 1999; 38: 1246–53.

Loney J, Milrich R. Hyperactivity, inattention, and aggression in clinical practice. In M Wolraich and DK Routh (eds). Advances in Developmental and Behavioral Pediatrics. Greenwich, CT: JAI Press, 1982: Vol 3; pp 113–47.

Pelham WE, Milich R, Murphy DA, Murphy HA. Normative data on the IOWA Conners Teacher Rating Scale. J Clin Child Psychol 1989; 18: 259–62.

Address

Jan Loney
Lodge Associates (Box 9)
Mayslick, KY 41055
USA
janloney@medscape.com

IOWA Conners Teacher's Rating Scale (IOWA Conners)

	Not at all	Just a little	Pretty much	Very much
1. Fidgeting (I/O)	0	1	2	3
2. Humans and makes odd noises (I/O)	0	1	2	3
3. Excitable, impulsive (I/O)	0	1	2	3
4. Inattentive, easily distracted (I/O)	0	1	2	3
5. Fails to finish things he/she starts, short attention span (I/O)	0	1	2	3
6. Quarrelsome (O/D)	0	1	2	3
7. Acts 'smart' (O/D)	0	1	2	3
8. Temper outbursts (explosive and unpredictable behavior) (O/D)	0	1	2	3
9. Defiant (O/D)	0	1	2	3
10. Uncooperative (O/D)	0	1	2	3

Note: Teachers score each problem as an average for the past 1 week. I/O = Inattention/Overactivity subscale; O/D = Oppositional/Defiant subscale.

Swanson, Kotkin, Atkins, M-Flynn, and Pelham Rating Scale (SKAMP)

Time 5 minutes

Ages 6–12

Time Frame Current observations in classroom

Purpose Assessment of ADHD problems.

Commentary

The SKAMP was developed to evaluate target behaviors specified in a school-based modification program. Attention problems which lead to decreased academic productivity and deportment problems which lead to classroom disruptions were selected as target behaviors.

Versions

The Swanson, Kotkin, Atkins, M-Flynn, and Pelham (SKAMP) rating scale is to be completed by teachers or observers.

Properties

Items   The SKAMP comprises 10 items that are rated on a 4-point scale indicating impairment with responses: not at all, just a little, quite a bit, and very much. However, other versions of the SKAMP exist in which the response scale is modified or items are added.

Scales   Factor analysis supported two factors, so the items of the SKAMP are scored on two subscales which are labeled Deportment and Attention.

Reliability   Test–retest correlations across two assessment sessions on one day in a clinical trial ranged from 0.63 to 0.78 for a placebo group and ranged from 0.21 to 0.75 for an experimental group.

Cronbach's alphas were 0.85 for Deportment, and 0.95 for Attention among elementary school children.

Validity   Correlations of the SKAMP with teacher-reported symptoms of ADHD ranged from 0.77 to 0.83 for Deportment and from 0.37 to 0.76 for Attention

among children in a clinical trial in which they were assessed several times. Associations with teacher-reported inattention were higher for Attention than for Deportment and associations with teacher-reported hyperactivity and impulsivity were higher for Deportment than for Attention in a sample of elementary school children.

Norms   A table with means and standard deviations for elementary school children aged 10 years, separate for boys and girls, is given in Swanson (1992).

Use   The SKAMP can be downloaded from the website at the address below.

Key references

McBurnett K, Swanson JM, Pfiffner LJ, Tamm L. A measure of ADHD related classroom impairment based on targets for behavioral intervention. J Atten Disord 1997; 2: 69–76.

Swanson JM. School-based assessment and interventions for ADD students. Irvine, CA: K. C. Publishing, 1992.

Swanson JM, Gupta S, Williams L, et al. Efficacy of a new pattern of delivery of methylphenidate for the treatment of ADHD: effects on activity level in the classroom and on the playground. J Am Acad Child Adolesc Psychiatry 2002; 41: 1306–14.

Wigal SB, Gupta S, Guinta D, Swanson JM. Reliability and validity of the SKAMP rating scale in a laboratory school setting. Psychopharmacol Bull 1998; 34: 47–53.

Address

James M. Swanson
University of California at Irvine
Child Development Center
Irvine, California 92612
USA
jmswanso@uci.edu
www.adhd.net

Swanson, Nolan, and Pelham-IV (SNAP-IV)

Time 15 minutes

Ages 6–12

Time Frame Not specified

Purpose Assessment of ADHD problems.

Commentary

The initial version SNAP (Swanson et al., 1980) was developed to assess ADHD symptoms, directly taken from the DSM-III. To ensure compatibility with the DSM, the SNAP was revised with each revision of the DSM. The SNAP-IV corresponds to the DSM-IV. In addition to the items for the DSM-IV ADHD criteria, the SNAP-IV also includes criteria for other disorders. However, many users of the SNAP-IV only select the ADHD and ODD items in their studies.

Versions

The Swanson, Nolan, and Pelham-IV (SNAP-IV) is available as a parent-report and a teacher report.

Properties

Items   The SNAP-IV comprises 90 items that are rated on a 4-point scale with responses: not at all, just a little, quite a bit, and very much. Items pertaining to AHDH are adapted from the 18 DSM-IV criteria for ADHD: 9 items pertaining to inattention, and 9 items pertaining to hyperactivity and impulsivity. The SNAP-IV also contains items taken from other rating scales to assess symptoms of ADHD, ODD, and conduct disorder. In addition, the SNAP-IV includes several items that assess symptoms of other DSM-IV disorders to screen for comorbid disorders.

Scales   The items of the SNAP-IV are scored on 9 subscales: ADHD-In indicates inattention problems, ADHD-H/Im indicates hyperactivity and impulsivity problems, ADHD-C is the combination of ADHD-In and ADHD-H/Im, ODD indicates oppositional defiant problems, I/O indicates inattention and overactivity, A/D indicates aggression and defiance, Conners Index indicates a general index of childhood problems, and Academic and Deportment indicate impairment in classroom settings.

Reliability   Cronbach's alphas were 0.76, 0.67, and 0.78 for teacher ratings of the ADHD-In, ADHD-H/Im, and ODD subscales, respectively among elementary school children.

Validity   In a clinical drug trial scores on ADHD-In, ADHD-H/Im, and ODD subscales decreased significantly in the two drug condition groups, but not in the placebo group.

Norms   The scoring instructions include cut-off scores for the ADHD-In, ADHD-H/Im, ADHD-C, and ODD subscales separately for teacher and parent ratings. However, no information is available on how these cut-off scores were obtained.

Use   The SNAP-IV and its scoring instructions can be downloaded from the website at the address below.

Key references

Stevens J, Quittner AL, Abikoff H. Factors influencing elementary school teacher's ratings of ADHD and ODD behaviors. J Clin Child Psychol 1998; 27: 559–65.

Swanson JM. School-based assessment and interventions for ADD students. Irvine, CA: K. C. Publishing, 1992.

Swanson JM, Nolan W, Pelham WE. SNAP rating scale. Educational Resources in Education, ERIC, 1982.

Wolraich ML, Greenhill LL, Pelham W, et al. Randomized, controlled trial of oros methylphenidate once a day in children with attention-deficit/hyperactivity disorder. Pediatrics 2001; 108: 883–992.

Address

James M. Swanson
University of California at Irvine
Child Development Center
Irvine, California 92612
USA
jmswanso@uci.edu
www.adhd.net

Vanderbilt ADHD Diagnostic Parent Rating Scale (VADPRS) and Vanderbilt ADHD Diagnostic Teacher Rating Scale (VADTRS)

Time 10 minutes

Ages VADPRS: 6–11; VADTRS: 6–12

Time Frame Not specified

Purpose Assessment of disruptive problems.

Commentary

The VADPRS and VADTRS were designed to assess disruptive problems modeled on DSM-IV criteria. All 18 criteria for ADHD are present in the scales.

Versions

The Vanderbilt ADHD Diagnostic Parent Rating Scale (VADPRS) is a rating scale to be completed by parents and the Vanderbilt ADHD Diagnostic Teacher Rating Scale (VADTRS) is a rating scale to be completed by teachers.

Properties

Items   The VADPRS comprises 47 items and the VADTRS 35 items. The items represent predominantly DSM-IV criteria for ADHD, but items representing DSM-criteria for oppositional defiant disorder, conduct disorder, anxiety and depression are included as well. The items are rated on a 4-point scale with responses never, occasionally, often, and very often. In addition, both scales include 8 performance items that are rated on a 5-point scale with only three labels: problematic, average, and above average.

Scales   Factor analysis was used to determine the structure of the items. For both scales a 4–factor structure was adequate. The items of the VADPRS and VADTRS are scored on 4 scales that are labeled: ADHD Inattentive type, ADHD hyper/impulsive type, ODD-CD, and Anxiety/depression. The performance items are scored on two scales labeled: Academic performance and Classroom Behavior Performance.

Reliability   Cronbach's alphas for the VADPRS scales were all above 0.90 for the 18 ADHD was 0.91 for ODD-CD, and was 0.79 for Anxiety/depression. Cronbach's alphas for the VADPRS scales were above 0.90 for the ADHD scales, 0.87 for OCC-CD, 0.80 for Anxiety/depression, 0.95 for Academic Performance, and 0.94 for Classroom Behavior Performance.

Validity   The VADPRS ADHD scale correlated significantly with ADHD ratings obtained with a diagnostic interview, and the ODD-CD and Anxiety/depression scales correlated significantly with impairment ratings. The VADTRS ADHD scales correlated significantly with ADHD diagnosis

Norms   Tables with means and standard deviations for the VADTRS scale scores of 10 056 ratings of 6–12–year-old children in elementary schools as well as tables with cutoff values for several cutpoints are given in Wolraich et al. (1998).

Use   No supplemental materials available.

Key references

Wolraich ML, Feurer ID, Hannah JN, Baumgaertel A, Pinnock TY. Obtaining systematic Teacher reports of disruptive disorders utilizing DSM-IV. J Abnorm Child Psychol 1998; 26: 141–52.

Wolraich ML, Lambert W, Doffing MA, et al. Psychometric Properties of the Vanderbilt ADHD Diagnostic Parent Rating Scale in a referred population. J Pediatr Psychol 2003; 28: 559–68.

Address

Mark L. Wolraich
OU Health Sciences Center
Child Study Center
1100 NE 13th Street
Oklahoma City, Oklahoma 73117
USA
mark-wolraich@ouhsc.edu

Antisocial Process Screening Device (APSD) – sample items

		Not at all true	Sometimes true	Definitely true
4.	Acts without thinking of the consequences	NT	ST	DT
10.	Uses or cons other people to get what he wants	NT	ST	DT
19.	Does not show feelings or emotions	NT	ST	DT

Children's Aggression Scale (CAS)

Time 10 minutes

Ages CAS-P: 7–11; CAS-T: 6–12

Time Frame Last year

Purpose Assessment of aggressive behaviors.

Commentary

The CAS-P and CAS-T were modeled on the Overt Aggression Scale (OAS; Yudofsky et al, 1986) an observational scale designed for adults.

Versions

The Children's Aggression Scales comprises two versions: the Children's Aggression Scale-Parent Version (CAS-P) to be completed by parents and the Children's Aggression Scale-Parent Version (CAS-T) to be completed by teachers.

Properties

Items The CAS-P comprises 33 items and the CAS-T 23 items. The items are rated on a 5-point scale with responses: never, once/month or less, once/week or less, 2–3 times/week, and most days or with responses: never, once a week, 3–5 times, 5–10 times, and more than 10 times. Both the CAS-P and CAS-T have one item rated on a 2-point scale with responses: yes, and no.

Scales The items of the CAS-P and CAS-T are scored on five subscales which are labeled: Verbal Aggression, Aggression Against Objects and Animals, Provoked Physical Aggression, Initiated Physical Aggression, and Use of Weapons.

Reliability Cronbach's alphas for the CAS-P ranged from 0.62 to 0.90 for the subscales and 0.93 for the entire CAS-P. Cronbach's alphas for the CAS-T ranged from 0.59 to 0.89 and 0.93 for the entire CAS-T.

Validity The CAS-P scales, except the Use of Weapons scale, correlated significantly with parent-rated measures of attention problems, aggressive behavior, and delinquent behavior. The CAS-P Verbal Aggression and Initiated Physical Aggression scales correlated significantly with teacher-reported measures of aggression and the scales did not correlate significantly with teacher-reported measures of inattention and overactivity. The CAS-T scales correlated significantly with parent-reported measures of aggressive and delinquent behavior, but not with attention problems. The CAS-T scales correlated significantly with teacher-reported measures of aggression and inattention and overactivity.

Among four diagnostic groups, the group with children diagnosed with conduct disorder had significantly higher scores on the CAS-T scales, except the Use of Weapons scale, than the children in the other groups who were diagnosed with oppositional defiant disorder, ADHD, or who had no ADHD or disruptive behavior disorder. The children with oppositional defiant disorder had higher scores on the CAS-P scales, except the Use of Weapons scale, than the children with ADHD and the children who had no ADHD or disruptive disorder. Among four diagnostic groups, the group with children diagnosed with conduct disorder had significantly higher scores on the CAS-T scales, except the Use of Weapons scale, than the children in the other groups who were diagnosed with oppositional defiant disorder, ADHD, or who had no ADHD or disruptive behavior disorder.

Norms Tables with means and standard deviations for the CAS-P subscale scores of 73 referred children can be found in Halperin et al. (2002). Tables with means and standard deviations for the CAS-T subscale scores of 67 referred children and 273 6–12-year-old children from elementary schools can be found in Halperin et al., (2003).

Use No supplemental materials available.

Key references

Halperin JM, McKay KE, Grayson RH, Newcorn JH. Reliability, validity, and preliminary normative data for the Children's Aggression Scale-Teacher Version. J Am Acad Child Adolesc Psychiatry 2003; 42: 965–71.

Halperin JM, McKay KE, Newcorn JH. Development, reliability, and validity of the Children's Aggression Scale-Parent Version. J Am Acad Child Adolesc Psychiatry 2002; 41: 245–52.

Yudofsky SC, Silver JM, Jackson, W, Endicott J, Williams D. The Overt Aggression Scale for the objective rating of verbal and physical aggression. Am J Psychiatry 1986; 143: 35–9.

Address

Jeffrey M. Halperin
Psychology Department
Queens College
65–30 Kissena Blvd.
Flushing, NY 11367
USA
e-mail: Jeffrey_halperin@qc.edu

Children's Aggression Scale (CAS) – Teacher Version

Child: _____ Gender: M F DOB: ___/___/___ Age: ____ Grade: ____ ID ____

School: _____ Respondent: _____ Relation to child: _____

I. VERBAL AGGRESSION: This section will focus on incidents in which there was no physical contact or fighting
DURING THE PAST YEAR, HOW OFTEN HAS THE ABOVE-NAMED CHILD:

1.	Snapped or yelled at other children?	Never	once/month or less	once/week or less	2–3 times/week	most days
2.	Snapped or yelled at adults?	Never	once/month or less	once/week or less	2–3 times/week	most days
3.	Cursed or sworn at other children?	Never	once/month or less	once/week or less	2–3 times/week	most days
4.	Cursed or sworn at adults?	Never	once/month or less	once/week or less	2–3 times/week	most days
5.	Verbally threatened to hit another child?	Never	once/month or less	once/week or less	2–3 times/week	most days
6.	Verbally threatened to hit an adult?	Never	once/month or less	once/week or less	2–3 times/week	most days

II. AGGRESSION AGAINST OBJECTS AND ANIMALS
DURING THE PAST YEAR, HOW OFTEN HAS THE ABOVE-NAMED CHILD:

7.	Slammed a door, kicked a chair or thrown or broken objects when angry?	Never	once/month or less	once/week or less	2–3 times/week	most days
8.	Intentionally vandalized or destroyed someone else's property?	Never	once/month or less	once/week or less	2–3 times/week	most days
9.	Taunted or teased or annoyed a pet or other animal?	Never	once/month or less	once/week or less	2–3 times/week	most days
10.	Injured or tortured a pet or other living animal?	Never	once or twice	3–5 times	5–10 times	more than 10 times

III. PHYSICAL AGGRESSION
A. PROVOKED PHYSICAL AGGRESSION – *this section will focus on instances where another person provoked or 'picked' a fight with the above-named child (i.e., when the other person made the first physical contact)*

DURING THE PAST YEAR, HOW OFTEN HAS THE ABOVE-NAMED CHILD:

11.	Fought with another child when provoked?	Never	once/month or less	once/week or less	2–3 times/week	most days
12.	Fought with an adult when provoked?	Never	once/month or less	once/week or less	2–3 times/week	most days
13.	How often did these fights result in mild physical injury (e.g., bumps and bruises)?	Never	once or twice	3–5 times	5–10 times	more than 10 times
14.	How often did these fights result in serious physical injury (e.g., stitches, broken bones, or requiring a doctor's attention)?	Never	once or twice	3–5 times	5–10 times	more than 10 times

Please describe:

B. INITIATED PHYSICAL AGGRESSION – *this section will focus on those fights which the above-named child initiated or started (i.e., when he/she made the first physical contact).*
DURING THE PAST YEAR, HOW OFTEN HAS THE ABOVE-NAMED CHILD:

15.	Started a physical fight with another child?	Never	once/month or less	once/week or less	2–3 times/week	most days
16.	Started a physical fight with an adult?	Never	once/month or less	once/week or less	2–3 times/week	most days
17.	How often did these fights result in mild physical injury (e.g., bumps and bruises)?	Never	once or twice	3–5 times	5–10 times	more than 10 times
18.	How often did these fights result in serious physical injury (e.g., stitches, broken bones, or requiring a doctor's attention)?	Never	once or twice	3–5 times	5–10 times	more than 10 times

Please describe:

IV. USE OF WEAPONS
DURING THE PAST YEAR, HOW OFTEN HAS THE ABOVE-NAMED CHILD:

19.	Carried a weapon (e.g., knife, gun)?	Never	once or twice	3–5 times	5–10 times	more than 10 times
20.	Threatened another with a weapon?	Never	once or twice	3–5 times	5–10 times	more than 10 times
21.	Used a weapon in a fight?	Never	once or twice	3–5 times	5–10 times	more than 10 times
22.	Injured another with a weapon?	Never	once or twice	3–5 times	5–10 times	more than 10 times
23.	Did this behavior occur only within the context of a gang?	YES	NO			

ADDITIONAL COMMENTS: _____

_____

_____

_____

_____

Children's Aggression Scale (CAS) – Parent Version

Child: _____ Gender: M F   DOB: ___/___/___ Age: ____ Grade: ____ ID ____

School:_____ Respondent:_____ Relation to child:_____

I. VERBAL AGGRESSION: *This section will focus on incidents in which there was no physical contact or fighting.*
DURING THE PAST YEAR, HOW OFTEN HAS YOUR CHILD:

1. Snapped or yelled at children living in the home?	Never	Once/month or less	Once/week or less	2–3 times/week	most days
2. Snapped or yelled at adults living in the home?	Never	Once/month or less	Once/week or less	2–3 times/week	most days
3. Snapped or yelled at peers/friends who do not live in the home?	Never	Once/month or less	Once/week or less	2–3 times/week	most days
4. Snapped or yelled at adults who do not live in the home?	Never	Once/month or less	Once/week or less	2–3 times/week	most days
5. Cursed or sworn at children who live in the home?	Never	Once/month or less	Once/week or less	2–3 times/week	most days
6. Cursed or sworn at adults who live in the home?	Never	Once/month or less	Once/week or less	2–3 times/week	most days
7. Cursed or sworn at peers/friends who do not live in the home?	Never	Once/month or less	Once/week or less	2–3 times/week	most days
8. Cursed or sworn at adults who do not live in the home?	Never	Once/month or less	Once/week or less	2–3 times/week	most days
9. Verbally threatened to hit a child who lives in the home?	Never	Once/month or less	Once/week or less	2–3 times/week	most days
10. Verbally threatened to hit an adult who lives in the home?	Never	Once/month or less	Once/week or less	2–3 times/week	most days
11. Verbally threatened to hit peers/friends who do not live in the home?	Never	Once/month or less	Once/week or less	2–3 times/week	most days
12. Verbally threatened to hit adults who do not live in the home?	Never	Once/month or less	Once/week or less	2–3 times/week	most days

II. AGGRESSION AGAINST OBJECTS AND ANIMALS
DURING THE PAST YEAR, HOW OFTEN HAS YOUR CHILD:

13. Slammed a door, kicked a chair, or thrown broken objects when angry?	Never	Once/month or less	Once/week or less	2–3 times/week	most days
14. Vandalized or destroyed someone else's property?	Never	Once/month or less	Once/week or less	2–3 times/week	most days
15. Taunted or teased or annoyed a pet or other animal?	Never	Once/month or less	Once/week or less	2–3 times/week	most days
16. Injured or tortured a pet or other living animal?	Never	Once/month or less	Once/week or less	2–3 times/week	most days

III. PHYSICAL AGGRESSION
A. PROVOKED PHYSICAL AGGRESSION – *this section will focus on instances where another person provoked or 'picked' a fight with your child (i.e., when the other person made the first physical contact).*
DURING THE PAST YEAR, HOW OFTEN HAS YOUR CHILD:

17. Fought with another child who lives in the home when provoked?	Never	Once/month or less	Once/week or less	2–3 times/week	most days
18. Fought with an adult who lives in the home when provoked?	Never	Once/month or less	Once/week or less	2–3 times/week	most days
19. Fought with peers/friends when provoked?	Never	Once/month or less	Once/week or less	2–3 times/week	most days
20. Fought with other adults who do not live in the home when provoked?	Never	Once/month or less	Once/week or less	2–3 times/week	most days
21. How often did these fights result in mild physical injury (e.g. bumps and bruises)	Never	Once/month or less	Once/week or less	2–3 times/week	most days
22. How often did these fights result in serious physical injury (e.g. stitches, broken bones, or requiring a doctor's attention)?	Never	Once/month or less	Once/week or less	2–3 times/week	most days

Please describe:_____

B. INITIATED PHYSICAL AGGRESSION – *this section will focus on those fights which your child initiated or started (i.e., when he/she made the first physical contact).*
DURING THE PAST YEAR, HOW OFTEN HAS YOUR CHILD:

23. Started a physical fight with a child who lives in the home?	Never	Once/month or less	Once/week or less	2–3 times/week	most days
24. Started a physical fight with an adult who lives in the home?	Never	Once/month or less	Once/week or less	2–3 times/week	most days

25. Started a physical fight with peers/friends who do not live in the home?	Never	Once/month or less	Once/week or less	2–3 times/week	most days
26. Started a physical fight with adults who do not live in the home?	Never	Once/month or less	Once/week or less	2–3 times/week	most days
27. How often did these fights result in mild physical injury (e.g. bumps and bruises)?	Never	Once or twice	3-5 times	5-10 times	more than 10 times
28. How often did these fights result in serious physical injury (e.g., stitches, broken bones, or requiring a doctor's attention)?	Never	Once or twice	3-5 times	5-10 times	more than 10 times

Please describe:_____

IV. USE OF WEAPONS
DURING THE PAST YEAR, HOW OFTEN HAS YOUR CHILD

29. Carried a weapon (e.g., knife, gun)?	Never	Once or twice	3-5 times	5-10 times	more than 10 times
30. Threatened another with a weapon?	Never	Once or twice	3-5 times	5-10 times	more than 10 times
31. Used a weapon in a fight?	Never	Once or twice	3-5 times	5-10 times	more than 10 times
32. Injured another with a weapon?	Never	Once or twice	3-5 times	5-10 times	more than 10 times
33. Did this behavior occur within the context of a gang?	YES	NO			

Children's Social Behavior Scale (CSBS) and Children's Social Behavior Scale-Teacher Form (CSBS-T)

Time 10 minutes

Ages 9–12

Time Frame Not specified

Purpose Assessment of social aggression.

Commentary

The CSBS was designed to assess types of aggressive behaviors that are specifically important to study social adjustment of children. The distinction between overt and relational aggression has been important for understanding gender differences in aggression.

Versions

The Children's Social Behavior Scale (CSBS) was initially designed as a peer nomination scale and subsequently adapted as a teacher scale (CSBS-T).

Properties

Items   The CSBS comprises 13 items. Children are asked to nominate up to three classmates for each item. CSBS-T comprises 15 items that are rated on a 5-point scale with responses from this is never true for this child to this is almost always true for this child.

Scales   The items of the CSBS are standardized within classrooms and the standardized items are summed to form three subscales. The items of the CSBS-T are scored on the same three subscales, but without standardization. The composition of three subscales is supported by factor analysis for both instruments. The subscales are: Overt Aggression, Relational Aggression, and Prosocial Behavior.

Reliability   Test–retest correlations across a 1-month interval ranged from 0.80 to 0.93 and across a 6 months interval ranged from 0.56 to 0.78 for Overt Aggression

and Relational Aggression in a sample of elementary-school children.

Cronbach's alphas were 0.94, 0.83, and 0.91 for peer nominations, and 0.94, 0.94, and 0.93 for teacher reports of Overt Aggression, Relational Aggression, and Prosocial Behavior, respectively in a sample of elementary-school children.

Validity   Peer-reported and teacher-reported Overt aggression are associated with peer rejection. Children classified as aggressive based on Relational Aggression reported more depressive symptoms, loneliness, peer isolation, and less peer acceptance than children classified as nonaggressive children.

Norms   No information available.

Use   A table with CSBS items is printed in Crick and Grotpeter (1995), and a table of CSBS-T items is printed in Crick (1996).

Key references

Crick NR. The role of overt aggression, relational aggression, and prosocial behaviour in the prediction of children's future social adjustment. Child Dev 1996; 67: 2317–27.

Crick NR, Grotpeter JK. Relational aggression, gender, and social-psychological adjustment. Child Dev 1995; 66: 710–20.

Address

Nicki R. Crick
Institute of Child Development
University of Minnesota
51 East River Road
Minneapolis, MN 55455–0345
USA
Crick001@umn.edu

Direct and Indirect Aggression Scale (DIAS)

Time 5 minutes

Ages 8–15

Time Frame Not specified

Purpose Assessment of aggression.

Commentary

The DIAS was designed to assess both direct and indirect aggression. Direct aggression, e.g. hitting and yelling, is overt and indirect aggression, e.g. gossiping and ignoring, is acted secretly so that the aggressor is unknown to the victim. Research findings confirmed the hypothesis that boys engage predominantly in direct aggression, while girls engage predominantly in indirect aggression.

Versions

The Direct and Indirect Aggression Scale (DIAS) is available as a peer report and a self-report.

Properties

Items   The DIAS comprises 24 items that are rated on 5-point scale with responses: never, seldom, sometimes, quite often, and very often.

Scales   The items of the DIAS are scored on 3 subscales which were supported by factor analysis. The 3 subscales are: Physical Aggression, Verbal Aggression, and Indirect Aggression.

Reliability   Cronbach's alphas ranged from 0.90 to 0.93 for Physical Aggression, from 0.88 to 0.92 for Verbal Aggression, and from 0.92 to 0.94 for Indirect Aggression of the peer-reported DIAS in samples of school children. For self-reports the ranges of Cronbach's alphas were, respectively 0.60 to 0.78, 0.65 to 0.69, and 0.69 to 0.84.

Validity   No information available.

Norms   No information available.

Use   The DIAS in several languages and its scoring instructions can be downloaded from the website at the address below.

Key references

Björkqvist K, Österman K, Kaukiainen A. The development of direct and indirect aggressive strategies in males and females. In: Björkqvist K, Niemelä P (eds.) Of Mice and Women: Aspects of Female Aggression. San Diego, CA: Academic Press, 1992: 51–64.

Österman K, Björkqvist K, Lagerspetz MJ, et al. Peer and self-estimated aggression and victimiation in 8–year-old children from five ethnic groups. Aggress Behav 1994; 20: 411–28.

Address

Kaj Björkqvist
Department of Developmental Psychology
Åbo Akademi University
P.O. Box 311, FIN-65101
Vasa
Finland
kaj.bjorkqvist@abo.fi
www.vasa.abo.fi/svf/up/dias.htm

Eyberg Child Behavior Inventory (ECBI) and Sutter-Eyberg Student Behavior Inventory-Revised (SESBI-R)

Time 10 minutes

Ages 2–16

Time Frame Current

Purpose Assessment of disruptive behavior.

Commentary

The ECBI exists since the early 1970s and was restandardized in 1999. The SESBI-R exists since the late 1980s and was revised in 1997.

Versions

The Eyberg Child Behavior Inventory (ECBI) is a rating scale to be completed by parents and the Sutter-Eyberg Student Behavior Inventory-Revised (SESBI-R) is a rating scale to be completed by teachers.

Properties

Items   The ECBI comprises 36 items and the SESBI-R 38 items that are rated on two scales: a 7-point scale that indicates how often behaviors occur and a yes-no scale that indicates whether the child's behavior is problematic.

Scales   The ECBI and SESBI-R are scored on two scales. The sum of all responses on the 7-point scale constitutes the Intensity scale and the number of yes responses on the yes-no scale constitutes the Problem scale.

Reliability   For the ECBI the test-retest correlations were 0.86 for the Intensity scale and 0.88 for the Problem scale across a 3-week interval, and 0.75 for both scales across a 10-month interval. For the SESBI-R the test-retest correlations were 0.87 for the Intensity scale and 0.93 for the Problem scale.

For the ECBI the Cronbach's alpha was 0.95 for the Intensity scale and the K-R 20 was 0.93 for the Problem scale. For the SESBI-R the Cronbach's alpha was 0.98 for the Intensity scale and the K-R 20 was 0.96 for the Problem scale.

Validity   Both scales of the ECBI correlated significantly with observational measures of child negative affect, nonacceptance, and dominance. Both scales also correlated significantly with internalizing and externalizing behavior assessed with other instruments, but the correlation with externalizing was significantly higher than the correlation with internalizing behavior. The scales did not correlate with observational measures of child positive affect. The scales of the ECBI discriminate between conduct-disordered and nonreferred children, among different diagnostic categories, between children in normal classes and in classes for exceptional student education.

The scales of the SESBI-R correlated significantly with observational measures of off-task and inappropriate behavior and did not correlate with noncompliance. The scales correlated highly with externalizing behavior and did not correlate or correlate only moderately with internalizing. The Intensity scale, but not the Problem scale discriminated between children in normal classes and in classes for exceptional student education assessed with other instruments.

Norms   The ECBI is standardized on a sample of 798 children from six outpatient settings. Raw scores are converted to T-scores. The manual also lists means and standard deviations of the scales for subgroups, including children with conduct-disordered behavior, children with chronic illness, children with developmental delays.

The SESBI-R is standardized on a sample of 415 elementary school children.

Use   A manual and rating scales are available from the publisher at the address below.

Key references

Eyberg S, Pincus D. ECBI & SESBI-R Eyberg Child Behavior Inventory and Sutter-Eyberg Student Behavior Inventory-Revised: Professional Manual. Lutz, Fl: Psychological Assessment Resources, Inc, 1999.

Funderburk BW, Eyberg SM, Rich BA, Behar L. Further psychometric evaluation of the Eyberg and Bahar rating scales for parents and teachers of preschoolers. Early Educ Dev 2003; 4: 67–81.

Querido JG, Eyberg SM. Psychometric properties of the Sutter-Eyberg Student Behavior Invetory-Revised with preschool children. Behav Ther 2003; 34: 1–15.

Querido JG, Warner TD, Eyberg SM. Parenting styles and child behavior in African American families of preschool children. J Clin Child Adolesc Psychol. 2002; 31: 272–7.

Rich BA, Eyberg SM. Accuracy of assessment: the discriminative and predictive powerof the Eyberg Child behaviour Inventory. Ambul Child Health 2001; 7: 249–57.

Address

Psychological Assessment Resources, Inc.
16204 N. Florida Avenue
Lutz, FL 33549
USA
www.parinc.com

Eyberg Child Behavior Inventory (ECBI) – sample items

| | | How often does this occur with your child? | | | | | | | | Is this a problem for you? |
		Never	Seldom		Sometimes		Often		Always		
10.	Acts defiant when doesn't get own way	1	2		3	4	5	6	7	YES	NO
29.	Interrupts	1	2		3	4	5	6	7	YES	NO

Home Situations Questionnaire (HSQ) and School Situations Questionnaire (SSQ)

Time 5 minutes

Time Frame Not specified

Ages HSQ: 4–11; SSQ: 6–11

Purpose Assessment of disruptive behavior.

Commentary

The HSQ and SSQ were designed to assess the pervasiveness and severity of children's disruptive behavior across multiple home and school situations.

Versions

The Home Situations Questionnaire (HSQ) is a questionnaire to be completed by parents and the School Situations Questionnaire (SSQ) is a questionnaire to be completed by teachers.

Properties

Items   The HSQ comprises 16 items and the SSQ 12 items that describe situations. For each item, informants first indicate whether a child presents problems with compliance to instructions, commands, or rules in these situations. These items are rated on a 2-point scale with response: yes and no. For each item responded to with yes the severity of that situation is rated on a 9-point scale ranging from mild to severe.

Scales   The items of HSQ and the SSQ are scored on two scales. The Number of Problem Settings is a count of the yes responses and the Mean Severity is the mean of the severity responses of the items with a yes response.

Reliability   Test–retest correlations ranged from 0.60 to 0.89 for the HSQ and from 0.63 to 0.82 for the SSQ across 14–28-day intervals. Cronbach's alphas ranged from 0.82 to 0.87 for the HSQ and from 0.89 to 0.91 for the SSQ.

Validity   The HSQ correlated significantly with similar scales from other instruments. Correlations ranged from 0.46 to 0.83 with scales indicating hyperactivity,

impulsivity, conduct problems, aggressive behavior or delinquent behavior.

Both the HSQ and SSQ discriminated significantly between children diagnosed with ADHD and normal children. Both scales were also sensitive to treatment in clinical trials evaluating the effects of Ritalin among children diagnosed with ADHD.

Norms   A table with means, standard deviations, and cut-off values indicating 1.5 standard deviation above the mean of HSQ ratings of 995 children and SSQ ratings of 599 children from the USA general population is given in Barkley and Murphy (1998). In addition, cutoff values for 1.5 standard deviation above the mean are given.

Use   The rating scales are printed in Barkley and Murphy (1998).

Key references

Altepeter TS, Breen MJ. The Home Situations Questionnaire (HSQ) and the School Situations Questionnaire (SSQ): normative data and an evaluation of psychometric properties. J Psychoeducational Assessment 1989; 7: 312–22.

Barkley RA, Esdelbrook C. Assessing situational variation in children's behavior problems: The Home and School Situations Questionnaires. In R. Prinz (Ed.), Advances in behavioral assessment of children and families. 1987; 3: 157–76.

Barkley RA, Murphy KR. Attention-Deficit Hyperactivity Disorder: A Clinical Workbook – Second Edition. New York: The Guilford Press, 1998.

Breen MJ, Altepeter TS. Factor structure of the Home Situations Questionnaire and the School Situation Questionnaire. J Pediatr Psychol 1991; 16: 50–67.

Address

Guilford Publications
72 Spring Street
New York, NY 10012
USA
www.guilford.com

New York Rating Scales (NYRS)

Time 15 minutes

Ages 3–17

Time Frame Past four weeks

Purpose Assessment of disruptive behaviors and positive peer relations.

Commentary

The NYRS assess symptoms relevant to DSM-IV diagnoses of oppositional defiant disorder and conduct disorder. In addition, the NYRS also assess peer relations which often accompany these disorders and predict negative outcome.

Versions

The New York Rating Scales (NYRS) comprise four forms: The New York Parent Rating Scale – Preschool-aged (NYPRS-P), the New York Teacher Rating Scale – Preschool-aged (NYTRS-P), the New York Parent Rating Scale – School-aged (NYPRS-S), and the New York Teacher Rating Scale – School-aged (NYTRS-S).

Properties

Items Both the preschool-aged forms comprise 38 items, the NYPRS-S 47, and the NYTRS-S 36 items. Most of the items pertain to disruptive behaviors, but the forms include two impairment items as well. All items are rated on a 4-point scale with responses: not at all, just a little, pretty much, and very much.

Scales Factor analysis was used to determine the factor structure of the scales. The items of the preschool-aged forms are scored on two subscales which are labeled Conduct Problems and Positive Peer Relations. The items of the school-aged forms are scored on four subscales which are labeled Defiance, Physical Aggression, Delinquency, and Positive Peer Relations. In addition, the school-aged forms include two composite scales as well, which are labeled the Antisocial Behavior Scale and the Conduct Problems Scale.

Reliability Test–retest correlations across a 6-month interval were 0.83 and 0.73 for the NYPRS-P and 0.40 and 0.72 for the NYTRS-P on Conduct Problems and Positive Peer Relations. Test–retest correlations across an 8-month interval ranged from 0.36 to 0.64 for the NYPRS-S and test-retest correlations across a 5-week interval ranged from 0.62 to 0.87 for the NYTRS-S.

Cronbach's alphas were 0.85 and 0.85 for the NYPRS-P, and 0.92 and 0.94 for the NYTRS-P on Conduct Problems and Positive Peer Relations in pre-kindergarten children. Cronbach's alphas ranged from 0.85 to 0.95 for the NYPRS-S in children who were at high risk for antisocial behavior and ranged from 0.73 to 0.96 for the NYTRS-S in school children.

Validity Scores on the Delinquency subscale and the Antisocial Behavior Scale of the NYPRS-S were significantly higher for adjudicated high-risk children than for non-adjudicated high-risk children. Scores on all subscales and composite scales of the NYTRS-S were significantly higher for children diagnosed with conduct disorder than for school children.

Norms Normative data for the NYTRS-S are available on 1258 school children in grades 1–10. A table with means and standard deviations for the NYTRS-S subscales can be found in Miller et al. (1995). Normative data for the preschool-aged forms are available for 159 children in pre-kindergarten programs.

Use The scales and normative data can be obtained from Laurie Miller Brotman at the address below.

Key references

Brotman LM, Dawson-McClure S, Gouley KK, et al. Older siblings benefit from a family-based prevention program for preschoolers at risk for conduct problems. J Fam Psychol 2005; 19: 581–91.

Brotman LM, Kamboukos D, Theise R. Symptom-specific measures for disorders usually first diagnosed in infancy, childhood or adolescence. In American Psychiatric Association. Task Force for the Handbook of Psychiatry Measures, eds. Handbook of Psychiatric Measures, 2nd edn. American Psychiatric Association (in press).

Ensink K, Robertson BA, Zissis C, Leger P, de Jager W. Conduct disorder among children in an informal settlement. Evaluation of an intervention programme. SA Med J 1997; 87: 1533–7.

Miller LS, Klein RG, Piacentini J, et al. The New York Rating Scale for disruptive and antisocial behavior. J Am Acad Child Adolesc Psychiatry 1995; 34: 359–70.

Address

Laurie Miller Brotman
Institute for Prevention Science
New York University Child Study Center
215 Lexington Avenue, 14th Floor
New York, NY 10016
USA
laurie.brotman@nyumc.org

New York Teacher Rating Scale (NYTRS) – sample items

Defiance subscale
    Defiant
    Breaks school rules
    Loses temper
Physical aggression subscale
    Acts violently to other children or adults
    Starts physical fights
    Assaults others

Delinquent aggression subscale
    Carries a knife or other weapon
    Has mugged someone
    Has used a knife or other weapon in a fight
Peer relations subscale
    Shows remorse when does something wrong
    Helpful to others
    Has at least one good friend

Proactive and Reactive Aggression Scale (PRA)

Time 1 minute

Ages Grades 1–6

Time Frame Not specified

Purpose Assessment of aggressive behavior.

Commentary

The PRA scale is a very short scale and therefore easy to complete by teachers for each child in their classroom. The items were carefully selected to ensure an optimal distinction between proactive and reactive aggression.

Versions

The Proactive and Reactive Aggression Scale (PRA) is only available as a teacher report.

Properties

Items The PRA scale comprises 6 items that are rated on a 5-point scale with responses never, and almost always at the extremes.

Scales Factor analysis supported two factors of each three items. The items of the PRA scale are scored on two subscales that are labeled: Proactive Aggression and Reactive Aggression.

Reliability Cronbach's alphas were 0.91 and 0.87 for Proactive Aggression, and 0.90 and 0.88 for Reactive Aggression in two samples of school children.

Validity The Proactive Aggression subscale correlated significantly with observer-reported proactive aggression, even when the Reactive Aggression subscale was partialled out and likewise, the Reactive Aggression subscale correlated significantly with observer-reported overreactive aggression, even when the Proactive Aggression subscale was partialled out.

Children were classified according to the Proactive Aggression and Reactive Aggression subscales into five subgroups consisting of proactive but not reactive aggressive children, reactive but not proactive aggressive children, both proactive and reactive aggressive children, rejected but not aggressive children, and non-aggressive children. The three groups with aggressive children had significantly higher peer-nominated aggression scores than the two groups with non-aggressive children.

Norms Normative data are not available.

Use No supplementary materials or information are available.

Key references

Dodge KA, Coie JD. Social-information-processing factors in reactive and proactive aggression in children's peer groups. J Pers Soc Psychol 1987; 53: 1146–58.

Address

Kenneth A. Dodge
Center for Child and Family Policy
Box 90264
Duke University
Durham, NC 27708
USA
dodge@duke.edu

Reactive and Proactive Aggression Scale (PRA)

Instructions: For each of the six statements, please fill in the oval of that number that *best applies* to this child.

		This situation is never true for this child	This situation is rarely true for this child	This situation is sometimes true for this child	This situation is usually true for this child	This situation is almost always true for this child
1.	When this child has been teased or threatened, he or she gets angry easily and strikes back	①	②	③	④	⑤
2.	This child always claims that other children are to blame in a fight and feels that they started the trouble	①	②	③	④	⑤
3.	When a peer accidentally hurts this child (such as by bumping into him or her), this child assumes that the peer meant to do it, and then overreacts with anger/fighting	①	②	③	④	⑤
4.	This child gets other kids to gang up on a peer that he or she does not like	①	②	③	④	⑤
5.	This child uses physical force (or threatens to use force) in order to dominate other kids	①	②	③	④	⑤
6.	This child threatens or bullies others in order to get his or her own way	①	②	③	④	⑤

3.10 Substance Abuse

Adolescent Alcohol and Drug Involvement Scale (AADIS)

Time 10 minutes

Ages 11–17

Time Frame Not specified

Purpose Assessment of alcohol and drug involvement.

Commentary

The AADIS is based on the Adolescent Alcohol Involvement Scale (AAIS; Mayer and Filstead, 1979) and the Adolescent Drug Involvement Scale (Moberg, 1983), thus combining alcohol and drug use problems in one scale, while preserving the scoring structure of the original scales. Its item wording and drug names were also updated to current terminology. The AADIS was designed to provide a short screen which determines the need for a full assessment of an adolescent's use of alcohol and drugs.

Versions

The Adolescent Alcohol and Drug Involvement Scale (AADIS) can by administered as an interview, but is available as a self-report form as well.

Properties

Items   The AADIS consists of two sections. The first section comprises 16 items pertaining to alcohol and drug use history that are rated on a 8-point scale with responses: never used, tried but quit, several times a year, several times a month, weekends only, several times a week, daily, and several times a day. The second section comprises 14 items pertaining to alcohol and drug involvement that are rated on 5- to 8-point scales with responses that are unique for each question. For example, the item 'Whom do you drink or use drugs with?' has responses: with parents or adult relatives, with brothers or sisters, with friends or relatives own age, with older friends, and alone.

Scales   Only the items of the first section of the AADIS are scored on the total score which is a weighted sum of the item ratings.

Reliability   Cronbach's alpha was 0.94 for the total score among adolescents from correctional institutions.

Validity   The AADIS discriminated between adolescents diagnosed with and without substance use disorder with a sensitivity of 0.62 and a specificity of 0.95.

Norms   Optimal cut points for the classification of substance use disorder among adolescents from correctional institutions are given in Winters et al. (2001).

Use   Copies of the interview and survey versions of the AADIS, and a manual can be downloaded from the website listed below.

Key references

Mayer J, Filstead WJ. The Adolescent Alcohol Involvement Scale: An instrument for measuring adolescents' use and misuse of alcohol. J Stud Alcohol 1979; 40: 291–300.

Moberg DP. The Adolescent Drug Involvement Scale. J Adolesc Chem Depend 1991; 2: 75–88.

Moberg DP. Screening for alcohol and other drug problems using the Adolescent Alcohol and Drug Involvement Scale (AADIS). Retrieved September 8 2005 from http://www.pophealth.wisc.edu/chppe/adis/.

Winters KC, Botzet A, Anderson N, Bellehumeur T, Egan B. Screening and assessment study. Retrieved September 8 2005 from http://www.pophealth.wisc.edu/chppe/adis/.

Address

D. Paul Moberg
Center for Health Policy and Program Evaluation
Department of Population Health Sciences
University of Wisconsin-Madison
502 North Walnut Street – Room 109
Madison, WI 53705–2335
USA
dpmoberg@wisc.edu
www.pophealth.wisc.edu/chppe/adis

Adolescent Alcohol and Drug Involvement Scale (AADIS)

COVER SHEET – TO BE COMPLETED BY STAFF

Name _____   ID# _____

DOB _____   Date _____

Age:

Sex: 1. Male
         2. Female

Ethnicity:

         1. African American
         2. Asian
         3. Caucasian/European American
         4. Hispanic
         5. Native American Indian
         6. OTHER:_____

Home Community:_____

Reason for Screening:_____

AADIS SCORING RESULTS

Items 1–14 are scored. (The weights assigned are basically the same as those originally used on the AAIS.) For each item 1–14, add the weights associated with the highest category circled [weights are the numbers in square brackets on the interview version]. If more than one answer is circled, use the highest. The higher the total score, the more serious the level of alcohol/drug involvement.

AADIS SCORE: _____ (Score of 37 or above suggests need for a full professional substance abuse assessment)

DO YOU RECOMMEND FULL ASSESSMENT (Regardless of the AADIS score)?
   0. NO
   1. YES

COMMENTS:

Screened By: _____

A. DRUG USE HISTORY

For each drug listed, please circle one number under the category that best describes your use pattern. If you are currently in residential treatment or secure custody, please answer regarding how often you typically used it, before you entered treatment or were taken into custody. Consider only drugs taken without prescription from your doctor; for alcohol, don't count just a few sips from someone else's drink.

	Never used	Tried but quit	Several times a year	Several times a month	Weekends only	Several times a week	Daily	Several times a day
Smoking tobacco (cigarettes, cigars)	0	1	2	3	4	5	6	7
Alcohol (beer, wine, liquor)	0	1	2	3	4	5	6	7
Marijuana or hashish (weed, grass, blunts)	0	1	2	3	4	5	6	7
LSD, MDA, mushrooms peyote, other hallucinogens (ACID, shrooms)	0	1	2	3	4	5	6	7
Amphetamines (speed, ritalin, ecstasy, crystal)	0	1	2	3	4	5	6	7
Powder cocaine (coke, blow)	0	1	2	3	4	5	6	7
Rock cocaine (crack, rock, freebase)	0	1	2	3	4	5	6	7
Barbiturates, (quaaludes, downers, ludes, blues)	0	1	2	3	4	5	6	7
PCP (angel dust)	0	1	2	3	4	5	6	7
Heroin, other opiates (smack, horse, opium, morphine)	0	1	2	3	4	5	6	7
Inhalants (glue, gasoline, spray cans, whiteout, rush, etc.)	0	1	2	3	4	5	6	7
Valium, Prozac, other tranquilizers (without Rx)	0	1	2	3	4	5	6	7
OTHER DRUG _____	0	1	2	3	4	5	6	7

B. AADIS

These questions refer to your use of alcohol and other drugs (like marijuana/weed or cocaine/rock). If you are currently in residential treatment or in custody, please answer regarding the time you were living in the community before you started treated or were taken into custody. Circle the answers which describe your use of alcohol and/or other drug(s). Even if none of the answers seem exactly right, please pick the ones that come closest to being true. If a question doesn't apply to you, you may leave it blank.

1. How often do you use alcohol or other drugs (such as weed or rock)?
   a. never
   b. once or twice a year
   c. once or twice a month
   d. every weekend
   e. several times a week
   f. every day
   g. several times a day

2. When did you last use alcohol or drugs?
   a. never used alcohol or drugs
   b. not for over a year
   c. between 6 months and 1 year before
   d. several weeks before
   e. the last week before
   f. the day before
   g. the same day I was taken into custody

3. I usually start to drink or use drugs because: (CIRCLE ALL THAT APPLY)
   a. I like the feeling
   b. to be like my friends
   c. I am bored; or just to have fun ('kickin' it')
   d. I feel stressed, nervous, tense, full of worries or problems
   e. I feel sad, lonely, sorry for myself

4. What do you drink, when you drink alcohol?
   a. wine
   b. beer
   c. mixed drinks
   d. hard liquor (vodka, whisky, etc.)
   e. a substitute for alcohol

5. How do you get your alcohol or drugs? (CIRCLE ALL THAT YOU DO)
   a. Supervised by parents or relatives
   b. from brothers or sisters
   c. from home without parents' knowledge
   d. get from friends
   e. buy my own (on the street or with false ID)

6. When did you first use drugs or take your first drink? (CIRCLE ONE)
   a. never
   b. after age 15
   c. at ages 14 or 15
   d. at ages 12 or 13
   e. at ages 10 or 11
   f. before age 10

7. What time of day do you use alcohol or drugs? (CIRCLE ALL THAT APPLY TO YOU)
   a. at night
   b. afternoons/after school
   c. before or during school or work
   d. in the morning or when I first awaken
   e. I often get up during my sleep to use alcohol or drugs

8. Why did you take your first drink or first use drugs? (CIRCLE ALL THAT APPLY)
   a. curiosity
   b. parents or relatives offered
   c. friends encouraged me; to have fun
   d. to get away from my problems
   e. to get high or drunk

9. When you drink alcohol, how much do you usually drink?
   a. 1 drink
   b. 2 drinks
   c. 3–4 drinks
   d. 5–9 drinks
   e. 10 or more drinks

10. Whom do you drink or use drugs with? (CIRCLE ALL THAT ARE TRUE OF YOU)
    a. parents or adult relatives
    b. with brothers or sisters
    c. with friends or relatives own age
    d. with older friends
    e. alone

11. What effects have you had from drinking or drugs? (CIRCLE ALL THAT APPLY TO YOU)
    a. loose, easy feeling
    b. got moderately high
    c. got drunk or wasted
    d. became ill
    e. passed out or overdosed
    f. used a lot and next day didn't remember what happened

12. What effects has using alcohol or drugs had on your life? (CIRCLE ALL THAT APPLY)
    a. none
    b. has interfered with talking to someone
    c. has prevented me from having a good time
    d. has interfered with my school work
    e. have lost friends because of use
    f. has gotten me into trouble at home
    g. was in a fight or destroyed property
    h. has resulted in an accident, an injury, arrest, or being punished at school for using alcohol or drugs

13. How do you feel about your use of alcohol or drugs? (CIRCLE ALL THAT APPLY)
    a. no problem at all
    b. I can control it and set limits on myself
    c. I can control myself, but my friends easily influence me
    d. I often feel bad about my use
    e. I need help to control myself
    f. I have had professional help to control my drinking or drug use

14. How do others see you in relation to your alcohol or drug use? (CIRCLE ALL THAT APPLY)
    a. can't say or normal for my age
    b. when I use I tend to neglect my family or friends
    c. my family or friends advise me to control or cut down on my use
    d. my family or friends tell me to get help for my alcohol or drug use
    e. my family or friends have already gone for help about my use

---

Developed by D. Paul Moberg, Center for Health Policy and Program Evaluation, University of Wisconsin Medical School. Adapted with permission from Mayer and Filstead's 'Adolescent Alcohol Involvement Scale' (Journal of Studies on Alcohol 40: 291–300, 1979) and Moberg and Hahn's 'Adolescent Drug Involvement Scale' (Journal of Adolescent Chemical Dependency, 2: 75–88, 1991).

Adolescent Substance Abuse Subtle Screening Inventory-Second Version (SASSI-A2)

Time 15 minutes

Ages 12–18

Time Frame One out of four time frames can be selected for items that assess frequency of alcohol and drug use: entire life, past six months, six months before a specified date, and six months since a specified date.

Purpose Assessment of substance use problems.

Commentary

The SASSI-A2 is a brief and easily administrated screening measure that helps identify individuals who have a high probability of having substance use disorder, i.e. substance abuse and substance dependence. The SASSI-A2 includes both face valid items and subtle items that are useful in identifying some adolescents who have a substance use disorder but are unable or unwilling to acknowledge the relevant behaviors. It is designed to help service providers determine if an adolescent is in need of further assessment and possible treatment for substance use disorders.

Versions

The Adolescent Substance Abuse Subtle Screening Inventory-Second Version (SASSI-A2) is only available as a self-report.

Properties

Items The SASSI-A2 comprises 28 items assessing frequency of alcohol and drug use that are rated on a 4-point scale with responses: never, once or twice, several times, and repeatedly. It also comprises 72 items consisting of items assessing associated symptoms, risks, and attitudes, and of subtle items that seem unrelated to substance use, but enable identifying people with substance problems even if they do not acknowledge substance misuse. These 72 items are rated on a 2-point scale with responses: true, and false. In addition, the SASSI-A2 comprises a few items that provide a brief history of an adolescent's substance use and legal problems.

Scales The items of the SASSI-A2 are scored on 12 subscales. The frequency items constitute two scales: Face Valid Alcohol (FVA), and Face Valid Other Drugs (FVOD). The true-false items constitute ten subscales. The first three, based on face valid items, are: Family-Friends Risk (FRISK); Attitudes (ATT), and Symptoms (SYM). Five subscales are based on items that seem unrelated to substance use: Obvious Attributes (OAT), Subtle Attributes (SAT), Defensiveness (DEF), Supplemental Addiction Measure (SAM), and Correctional (COR). In addition, the SASSI-A2 includes a validity check scale (VAL), and a Secondary Classification Scale (SCS) for differentiating between substance abuse and dependence.

Reliability Test–retest correlations across a 2-week interval ranged from 0.71 to 0.92 in a sample of clinical adolescents.

Cronbach's alphas ranged from 0.61 to 0.95 in a sample of clinical adolescents.

Validity In a sample of adolescents recruited from service settings the SASSI-A2 distinguished between adolescents diagnosed with a substance use disorder and those without a substance use disorder with a sensitivity of 95% and a specificity of 89%.

Norms The SASSI-A2 was standardized on ratings of 856 adolescents aged 12–18 years recruited from schools and community youth programs. Raw scores were converted to T-scores.

Use A manual, user's guide, rating scales, scoring key, scoring profiles, and a computer program can be obtained from the SASSI Institute at the address below.

Key references

Miller FG, Lazowski LE . The Adolescent SASSI-A2 Manual. Identifying Substance Use Disorders. Springville, IN: The SASSI Institute, 2001.

Miller FG, Lazowski LE. Substance Abuse Subtle Screening Inventory for Adolescents-Second Version. In Grisso T, Vincent G, Seagrave D (Eds.) Mental Health Screening and Assessment in Juvenile Justice. New York: The Guilford Press, 2005.

Miller FG, Renn WR, Lazowski LE. The Adolescent SASSI-A2 User's Guide. A Quick Reference for Administration and Scoring. Springville, IN: The SASSI Institute, 2001.

Address

The SASSI Institute
201 Camelot Lane
Springville, IN 47462
USA
www.sassi.com

For each item below, circle the number which reflects how often you have experienced the situation described during:

☐ your entire life   ☐ the six months before
☐ the past six months   ☐ the six months since

Karen K.

ALCOHOL (FVA)

	Never	Once or Twice	Several Times	Repeatedly
1. Drank alcohol during the day?	0	1	(2)	3
2. Taken a drink or drinks to help you talk about your feelings and ideas?	0	1	(2)	3
3. Taken a drink or drinks so you wouldn't feel tired or to give you a lift when you have to keep going?	0	1	(2)	3
4. Had more to drink than you intended to?	(0)	1	2	3
5. Gotten sick from drinking (e.g., vomiting, dizziness, headache)?	(0)	1	2	3
6. Gotten into trouble in school, at home, on the job, or with the police because of your drinking?	(0)	1	2	3
7. Become very sad or felt "down" after having sobered up?	(0)	1	2	3
8. Argued with your family or friends because of your drinking?	(0)	1	2	3
9. Had a strange experience when drinking (such as seeing something not really there) that came back again when you hadn't been drinking for a while?	(0)	1	2	3
10. Lost friends because of your drinking?	(0)	1	2	3
11. Felt really nervous or shaky after having sobered up?	(0)	1	2	3
12. Tried to kill yourself while drunk?	(0)	1	2	3

OTHER DRUGS (FVOD)*

*Does not include proper use of medications prescribed for you.

	Never	Once or Twice	Several Times	Repeatedly
1. Taken drugs to improve your thinking and feeling?		1	(2)	3
2. Taken drugs to help you feel better about a problem?		1	(2)	3
3. Taken drugs to be more aware of your senses (e.g., sight, hearing, touch, etc.)?	(0)	1	2	3
4. Taken drugs so you could enjoy sex more?	0	(1)	2	3
5. Taken drugs to help forget about feelings of being helpless or worthless?	0	1	2	3
6. Taken drugs to forget school, work, or family pressures?	(0)	1	(2)	3
7. Gotten into trouble in school, at home, on the job, or with the police because of your drug use?	(0)	1	2	3
8. Gotten really stoned or wiped out on drugs (more than just high)?	(0)	1	(2)	3
9. Tried to talk a doctor into giving you some prescription drug (e.g., tranquilizers, pain killers, diet pills)?	(0)	1	2	3
10. Spent your spare time in buying, selling, taking or talking about drugs?	(0)	1	2	3
11. Used alcohol and other drugs at the same time?	(0)	1	2	3
12. Continued to take a drug or drugs so you wouldn't feel physically uncomfortable or even sick from not having the drug(s)?	(0)	1	2	3
13. Felt your drug use has kept you from getting what you want out of life?	(0)	1	2	3
14. Been accepted into a treatment program because of your drug use?	(0)	1	2	3
15. Gone to school after drinking or using drugs?	(0)	1	2	3
16. Drank or used drugs away from home?	0	1	(2)	3

B1. Describe your current alcohol or drug use:
☐ More than twice a week   ☐ About twice a week   ☐ About once a week   ■ Between 1 and 3 times a month   ☐ Less than once a month   ☐ None

B2. How old were you when you first tried alcohol or drugs? ☐ 17   18   ☐ I've never tried alcohol or drugs.

B3. How old were you when you started using alcohol or drugs regularly? ☐ Less than 12   ☐ 12   ■ 13   ☐ 14   ☐ 15   ☐ 16   ☐ 17   ☐ 18   ■ I've never used regularly.

B4. Have your grades ever gone down due to your alcohol or drug use? ☐ Yes ☐ No ■ I've never used.

B5. a. Are you currently a student? ■ Yes ☐ No
    b. What is the highest grade you have completed? ☐ 5 ☐ 6 ☐ 7 ☐ 8 ☐ 9 ■ 10 ☐ 11 ☐ 12 ☐ Other _____

B6. Have you ever been in trouble with the law? ■ Yes ☐ No

the S·A·S·S·I

ADOLESCENT
SASSI-A2

Fill in this way □
Not like this ☑

If a statement is MOSTLY TRUE for you, fill in the box in the column headed "T" this way
If a statement is MOSTLY FALSE for you, fill in the box in the column headed "F" this way

T F

1. People will probably succeed if they work hard.
2. At least one of my parents has often been very sad, anxious, or unhappy.
3. I have never been in trouble with the principal or the police.
4. I can be friendly with people who do many wrong things.
5. I do not like to sit and daydream.
6. The school rules regarding getting caught with drugs are too strict.
7. Sometimes I have a hard time sitting still.
8. I have not lived the way I should.
9. I have had days, weeks, or months when I couldn't get much done because I just wasn't up to it.
10. I always listen carefully to people who are older than me.
11. I like to obey the rules.
12. I have often felt bad or scared because of the drinking or drug use of someone in my family.
13. Some crooks are so clever that I hope they don't get caught.
14. I have never done anything dangerous just for fun.
15. I am always well behaved in school.
16. I have sometimes drunk too much beer or other alcoholic drink.
17. Sometimes I wish I had better control of how I behave and feel.
18. Adults shouldn't hassle kids so much about drugs.
19. I break more rules than most people my age.
20. Swearing and cursing have become a serious problem in our schools and must be stopped.
21. I'm friends with some people who sell drugs.
22. I am usually happy.
23. I have been tempted to hit someone.
24. I always feel sure of myself.
25. My school teachers have had some problems with me.
26. Many of my friends drink or get high regularly.
27. I have never broken an important rule.
28. There have been times when I have done things I didn't remember later.
29. Getting caught drinking or using drugs is no big deal.
30. I think carefully about everything I do.
31. I have used alcohol or "pot" too much or too often.
32. Some of my friends have bad reputations.
33. I smoke cigarettes regularly.
34. At times I have been so full of energy that I felt I didn't need to sleep for days at a time.
35. Adults don't really know how much teenagers are using drugs.
36. I have never felt sad over anything.

T F

37. I think there is something wrong with my memory.
38. I have neglected schoolwork because of my drinking or drug use.
39. I have taken a drink in the morning to steady my nerves or to get rid of a hangover.
40. I often daydream about things that I don't tell other people.
41. I have wanted to run away from home.
42. People who use drugs have more fun.
43. I like doing things with my family.
44. It doesn't really bother me to see animals suffer.
45. At times I feel worn out for no reason at all.
46. I can see why they have laws about drugs like cocaine and heroin but outlawing marijuana is stupid.
47. No one has ever criticized or punished me.
48. I think carefully about how I dress.
49. My drinking or other drug use causes problems between me and my family.
50. I have skipped school pretty often.
51. Most of the people my age drink or use drugs.
52. Sometimes I like doing the opposite of what others want.
53. My parents like my friends.
54. In new situations I like to find out which people it would be useful to be friendly with.
55. One of my parents was/is a heavy drinker or drug user.
56. In school I have often been in trouble for misbehaving.
57. More often than not I have a sense that life is worthwhile.
58. I have used alcohol to excess.
59. When I'm in a group I have trouble thinking of the right things to talk about.
60. Drugs help people to be creative.
61. My grades in school are average or better.
62. I don't really worry about catching diseases.
63. Sometimes I feel that my drug use or drinking is keeping me from getting what I want out of life.
64. I've frequently played sick to get out of something.
65. I think many adults who say they are against drugs probably use some kind of drugs themselves.
66. My parents hardly ever know where I am.
67. My participation in clubs, sports, or other after school activities is important in my life.
68. I am often restless or jumpy.
69. I have sometimes just sat about when I should have been working.
70. The drug laws we have are stupid.
71. If some friends and I were in trouble together, I would rather take the whole blame than tell on them.
72. I can be depended on to do the things I am supposed to.

Name or Client ID _____ _Karen K._ Date _____

Sex M□ F■ Age □12 □13 □14 □15 □16■ □17 □18 □Other

Ethnicity: □African American □Asian American □Hispanic American □Native American □Caucasian □Mixed Race □Other

the S·A·S·S·I

Personal Experience Inventory (PEI)

Time 50 to 55 minutes for 12–15-year-olds; 45 to 50 minutes for 16–18-year-olds

Ages 12–18

Time Frame Most items have no specified time frame. Only items about drug history have three different specified time frames: lifetime, last 12 months, and last 3 months.

Purpose Assessment of drug involvement, accompanying psychosocial problems, and drug history.

Commentary

The PEI was developed to provide clinicians with a standardized self-report inventory to assist in the identification, referral, and treatment of problems associated with adolescent alcohol and drug abuse. It was not designed to provide a specific diagnosis of chemical dependency. The PEI is a combination of two separately developed rating scales: the Personal Experience With Chemicals Scale (PECS; Henly and Winters, 1988) and the Personal Experience Scales (PES; Henly and Winters, 1989).

Versions

The Personal Experience Inventory (PEI) was originally developed as a self-report form, but recent research provided support for a parent-completed form as well.

Properties

Items   The PEI comprises 300 items in two sections. The first section, Chemical Involvement Problem Severity, comprises 153 items pertaining to drug involvement and drug use. Most items of the first section are rated on a 4-point scale with responses: never, once or twice, sometimes, and often. A variety of response scales are used for other items in this section. For example, items pertaining to experiences are rated on a 2-point scale with responses: yes and no, and items pertaining to drug history are rated on a 7-point scale with responses: never, 1 or 2 times, 3 to 5 times, 6 to 9 times, 10 to 19 times, 20 to 39 times, and 40 or more times.

The second section, Psychosocial, comprises 147 items pertaining to personal en environmental risk factors. The items are rated on a 4-point scale with responses: strongly disagree, disagree, agree, and strongly agree; on a 4-point scale with responses: seldom or never, sometimes, often, and almost always; on a 3-point scale with responses: never, once or twice, and more than once or twice.

Scales   Since the PEI is a combination of two rating scales, the development of scales was conducted separately. The scales were developed using rational and empirical methods. Empirical methods include factor analysis, cluster analysis, and item response theory. The items of the first section are divided into five Basic Scales, five Clinical Scales, and three validity indices. Items on drug use frequency and duration, and items on age of onset are not organized into scales. The Basic Scales are: Personal Involvement With Chemicals, Effects From Drug Use, Social Benefits of Drug Use, Personal Consequences of Drug Use, and Polydrug Use. The five Clinical Scales are: Social-Recreational Drug Use, Psychological Benefits of Drug Use, Transsituational Drug Use, Preoccupation With Drugs, and Loss of Control. The three validity indices, pertaining to response distortion, are: Infrequency, Defensiveness, and Pattern Misfit. In addition, this section provides items on frequency, duration, and age of onset of drug use, but these items do not form scales.

The items of the second section are divided into eight Personal Risk Factors Scales, four Environmental Risk Factor Scales, and two validity indices. The Personal Risk Factors Scales are: Negative Self-Image, Psychological Disturbance, Social Isolation, Uncontrolled, Rejecting Convention, Deviant Behavior, Absence of Goals, and Spiritual Isolation. The Environmental Risk Factor Scales are: Peer Chemical Environment, Sibling Chemical Use, Family Pathology, and Family Estrangement. The validity indices are: Infrequency-2, and Defensiveness-2. In addition, several items from this section form brief screeners for the following problem areas: Need for Psychiatric Referral, Eating Disorder, Physical Abuse, Sexual Abuse, Family Chemical Dependency History, and Suicide potential.

Reliability   Test–retest correlations across a 1-week interval in a drug clinic sample ranged from 0.56 to 0.92 for the Chemical Involvement Problem Severity scales, from 0.40 to 0.89 for the Psychosocial scales, and from 0.38 to 0.58 for the validity indices. Test–retest correlations across a 1-month interval ranged from 0.50 to 0.84 for the Chemical Involvement Problem Severity scales, from 0.23 to 0.85 for the Psychosocial scales, and from 0.13 to 0.54 for the validity indices in drug clinic sample, from 0.44 to 0.90 for the Chemical Involvement Problem Severity scales, from 0.66 to 0.92 for the Psychosocial scales, and from 0.45 to 0.77 for the validity indices in a school sample. Test–retest kappas for brief screeners across a 1-week interval ranged from 0.34 to 0.74 in a drug clinic sample, across a 1-month interval ranged from 0.18 to 0.72 in a drug clinic sample, from 0.62 to 0.80 in a school sample.

Cronbach's alphas ranged from 0.87 to 0.97 for the Chemical Involvement Problem Severity scales, from 0.69 to 0.86 for the Psychosocial scales, and from 0.63 to 0.73 for the validity indices in a drug clinic sample, from 0.87 to 0.97 for the Chemical Involvement Problem Severity scales, from 0.66 to 0.90 for the Psychosocial scales, and from 0.65 to 0.79 for the validity indices in a juvenile offender sample, from 0.70 to 0.95 for the Chemical Involvement Problem Severity scales, from 0.70 to 0.90 for the Psychosocial scales, and from 0.53 to 0.75 for the validity indices in a school sample.

Validity   The Chemical Involvement Problem Severity scales correlated significantly and highly with alternate self-reported measures of alcohol and drug problem severity. The Psychosocial scales pertaining to personal and interpersonal adjustment correlated with self-reported multiple personality dimensions, but scales pertaining to values and characteristics of others did not. The validity indices correlated significantly with corresponding alternate measures of response distortion, with the exception of Infrequency-2 that was associated with self-reported defensiveness.

Scores on the Chemical Involvement Problem Severity scales, with the exception of two scales, were significantly higher for adolescents with a prior treatment history than for adolescents without prior treatment history in a drug clinic sample. Only one Psychosocial scale was significantly different in the expected direction between these adolescents. Scores on the Chemical Involvement Problem Severity scales and the Psychosocial scales were all significantly different among adolescents in a drug clinic sample, a juvenile offender sample, and a school sample.

Norms   The PEI was standardized on 1120 adolescents aged 12–18 years who were undergoing evaluation or treatment for chemical dependency and on 693 high school students in grades 7–12. Raw scores are converted to normalized T-scores.

Use

A manual and rating forms with multiple options for computer scoring are available from the publisher at the address below.

Key references

Henly GA, Winters KC. Development of problem severity scales for the assessment of adolescent alcohol and drug abuse. Int J Addict 1988; 23: 65–85.

Henly GA, Winters KC. Development of psychosocial scales for the assessment of adolescents involved with alcohol and drugs. Int J Addict 1989; 24: 973–1001.

Winters KC, Anderson N, Bengston P, Stinchfield RD, Latimer WW. Development of a parent questionnaire for use in assessing adolescent drug abuse. J Psychoactive Drugs 2000; 32: 3–13.

Winters KC, Stinchfield RD, Henly GA, Schwarz RH. Validity of adolescent self-report of alcohol and other drug involvement. Int J Addict 1990; 25: 1379–95.

Winters KC, Henly GA. Personal Experience Inventory (PEI): Manual. Los Angeles: Western Psychological Services, 1989.

Winters KC, Stinchfield RD, Henly GA. Further validation of new scales measuring adolescent alcohol and other drug abuse. J Stud Alcohol 1993; 54: 534–41.

Address

Western Psychological Services
12031 Wilshire Blvd.
Los Angeles, CA 90025–1251
USA
www.wpspublish.com

Personal Experience Inventory (PEI) – sample items

Part I

	Never	Once or twice	Sometimes	Often
How often have you used alcohol or other drugs:				
16. Soon after getting up in the morning	0	I	2	3
How often have you:				
36. Avoided family activities so you could get high	0	I	2	3
When using alcohol or other drugs, how often have you:				
53. Become depressed or really sad	0	I	2	3
In order to get or pay for alcohol or other drugs, how often have you:				
70. Borrowed money or gone into debt	0	I	2	3

	Never	Once or twice	More than once or twice
How many times have you:			
74. Gotten into fights with friends due to using drugs or alcohol	0	I	3+

	Yes	No
Please answer the following questions about your experiences:		
91. There have been times when I took advantage of someone	Y	N

	Never	Once or twice	Sometimes	Often
How often have you used each of these chemicals in order to get high:				
101. Marijuana (grass, pot) or Hashish (hash)	0	I	2	3

	Never	1 or 2 times	3 to 5 times	6 to 9 times	10 to 19 times	20 to 39 times	40 or more times
How many times (if any) have you used cocaine (sometimes called 'coke'):							
a. In your lifetime	O	O	O	O	O	O	O
b. During the last 12 months	O	O	O	O	O	O	O
c. During the last 3 months	O	O	O	O	O	O	O

	Never	Grade 6 or before	Grade 7 or 8	Grade 9 or 10	Grade 11 or after
How old were you when:					
124. You first got high on alcohol	O	O	O	O	O

Part II

	Strongly disagree	Disagree	Agree	Strongly agree
9. It would be better if I were dead	SD	D	A	SA
51. I'm afraid of someone in my family	SD	D	A	SA
70. It's important to have plans for the future	SD	D	A	SA

	Seldom or never	Sometimes	Often	Almost always
How often do these things happen:				
86. I feel guilty or ashamed	0	I	2	3
119. I get angry and lose my temper	0	I	2	3
126. I have a parent who hits me	0	I	2	3

	Never	Once or twice	More than once or twice
133. I have broken into a locked home or building	0	I	3+
147. I have been sexually abused by someone outside my family	0	I	3+

Personal Experience Screening Questionnaire (PESQ)

Time 10 minutes

Ages 12–18

Time Frame Most items have no specified time frame. Only a few items about drug history have a time frame that refers to the past 12 months.

Purpose Assessment of drug involvement, accompanying psychosocial problems, and drug history.

Commentary

The PESQ was designed as a brief screening tool to identify adolescents likely to need a drug abuse assessment referral. It is not intended to provide a formal diagnosis, but was constructed to indicate whether an adolescent should be referred for a comprehensive assessment. It assesses both alcohol and other drug involvement.

Versions

The Personal Experience Screening Questionnaire (PESQ) is only available as a self-report form.

Properties

Items The PESQ comprises 40 items in three parts. The first part comprises 21 items pertaining to drug use behaviours, experiences, and attitudes. Three of these items reflect faking-bad tendencies. The items in the first part are rated on a 4-point scale with responses: never, once or twice, sometimes, and often. The second part comprises 13 items pertaining to psychosocial problems and faking good tendencies. These items are rated on a 2-point scale with responses: yes and no. The third part comprises 6 items pertaining to the frequency of alcohol and drug use, hard drugs use, and drug use onset. The items on frequency of alcohol and drug use are rated on a 7-point scale with responses: never, 1–2 times, 3–5 times, 6–9 times, 10–19 times, 20–39 times, and 40+ times. The items on drug onset are rated on 5-point scale with responses: never, grade 6 or before, grade 7–8, grade 9–10, and grade 11 or after.

Scales Factor analysis was used to select the items for the subscale Problem Severity. In addition, two response tendency scales are derived: Infrequency indicates a faking-bad tendency and Defensiveness indicates a faking-

good tendency. The items on psychosocial problems and drug history are not scored on subscales, but provide supplemental information for clinical evaluation.

Reliability Cronbach's alphas for the Problem Severity subscale ranged from 0.90 to 0.91 in a drug clinic sample, from 0.93 to 0.95 in a juvenile offender sample, and from 0.90 to 0.92 in a normal school sample.

Validity The Problem Severity subscale correlated significantly with self-reported drug involvement, effects, social benefits, and personal consequences of drug use, and polydrug use.

Individuals with a prior treatment history had significantly higher Problem Severity scores than individuals without a treatment history, and individuals with a diagnosis of drug abuse had significantly higher scores than individuals with diagnosis of drug dependence in a drug clinic sample. Among three samples, the drug clinic sample had significantly higher scores than the juvenile offender sample and the normal school sample. In addition, the juvenile offender sample had significantly higher scores than the normal school sample.

Norms The PESQ is standardized on 646 individuals from drug clinics. Cutoff values are provided to determine whether an individual's score constitutes a clinical problem.

Use Rating forms which enable scoring and a manual are available from the publisher at the address below.

Key references

Winters KC. Personal Experience Screening Questionnaire (PESQ): Manual. Los Angeles: Western Psychological Services, 1991.

Winters KC. Development of an adolescent alcohol and other drug abuse screening scale: Personal Experience Screening Questionnaire. Addict Behav 1992; 17: 479–90.

Address

Western Psychological Services
12031 Wilshire Blvd.
Los Angeles, CA 90025–1251
USA
www.wpspublish.com

Personal Experience Screening Questionnaire (PESQ) – sample items

	Never	Once or twice	Sometimes	Often
How often have you used alcohol or other drugs:				
4. At the homes of friends or relatives	*	*	*	*
How often have you:				
11. Gotten drugs from a dealer	*	*	*	*

	Yes	No
Please answer the following questions about your experiences:		
23. I worry a lot about little things or for no reason	*	*

	Never	1–2 times	3–5 times	6–9 times	10–19 times	20–39 times	40+ times
During the past 12 months, how many times (if any):							
37. Have you used hard drugs other than alcohol or marijuana	*	*	*	*	*	*	*

Rutgers Alcohol Problem Index (RAPI)

Time 10 minutes

Ages 12–21

Time Frame Last year is recommended, but can be varied depending upon clinical or research goals

Purpose Assessment of problem drinking.

Commentary

The RAPI was designed to be a conceptually sound, unidimensional, brief, and easily administered instrument for the assessment of problem drinking in adolescence. It does not assess intensity of use, motivations for use, and contexts of use which may be desirable when a full assessment of problem drinking is desirable.

Versions

The Rutgers Alcohol Problem Index (RAPI) is only available as a self-report. Most people are currently using the 18-item shorter version instead of the 23-item original version.

Properties

Items   The RAPI comprises 18 or 23 items that are rated on a 4-point scale with response: none, 1-2 times, 3-5 times, and more than 5 times.

Scales   The RAPI consists only of a total score which is the sum of all items.

Reliability   Test–retest correlations were 0.83 across a 1-month interval, 0.86 across a 6-month interval, and 0.88 across a 1-year interval in a sample of undergraduate students.

Split-half reliability of the RAPI was 0.92 in a community sample.

Validity   The RAPI correlated significantly and above 0.70 with other measures of alcohol use and misuse in clinical samples. It discriminated between casual drinking and problem drinking in adolescents. The RAPI was sensitive to treatment in a clinical trial that evaluated a brief intervention designed to reduce harmful consequences of heaving drink among high-risk college students.

Norms   Tables with means and standard deviations separated by sex and age are available for clinical and nonclinical adolescents.

Use   The RAPI, a brief manual, and scoring instructions can be obtained from Helene White at the address below.

Key references

Marlatt GA, Baer JS, Kivlahan DR, et al. Screening and brief intervention for high-risk college student drinkers: results from a 2-year follow-up assessment. J Consult Clin Psychol 1998; 66: 604–15.

Miller ET, Neal DJ, Roberts LJ, et al. Test–retest reliabiity of alcohol measures: Is there a difference between internet-based assessment and traditional methods? Psychol Addict Behav 2002; 16: 56–63.

White HR, Labouvie EW. Toward the assessment of adolescent problem drinking. J Stud Alcohol 1989; 50: 30–7.

Address

Helene White
Center of Alcohol Studies
Rutgers University
Piscataway, NJ 08854-0969
USA
hewhite@rci.rutgers.edu

Rutgers Alcohol Problem Index (RAPI)

Different things happen to people while they are drinking ALCOHOL or because of their ALCOHOL drinking. Several of these things are listed below.
Indicate how many times each of these things happened to you WITHIN THE LAST YEAR.

Use the following code:

1 = None
    2 = 1–2 times
        3 = 3–5 times
            4 = More than 5 times

HOW MANY TIMES HAS THIS HAPPENED TO YOU WHILE YOU WERE DRINKING OR BECAUSE OF YOUR DRINKING DURING THE LAST YEAR?

1 2 3 4   Not able to do your homework or study for a test
1 2 3 4   Got into fights with other people (friends, relatives, strangers)
1 2 3 4   Missed out on other things because you spent too much money on alcohol

1 2 3 4   Went to work or school high or drunk
1 2 3 4   Caused shame or embarrassment to someone
1 2 3 4   Neglected your responsibilities

1 2 3 4   Relatives avoided you
1 2 3 4   Felt that you needed more alcohol than you used to in order to get the same effect
1 2 3 4   Tried to control your drinking (tried to drink only at certain times of the day or in certain places, that is, tried to change your pattern of drinking)

1 2 3 4   Had withdrawal symptoms, that is, felt sick because you stopped or cut down on drinking
1 2 3 4   Noticed a change in your personality
1 2 3 4   Felt that you had a problem with alcohol

1 2 3 4   Missed a day (or part of a day) of school or work
1 2 3 4   Wanted to stop drinking but couldn't
1 2 3 4   Suddenly found yourself in a place that you could not remember getting to

1 2 3 4   Passed out or fainted suddenly
1 2 3 4   Had a fight, argument or bad feeling with a friend
1 2 3 4   Had a fight, argument or bad feeling with a family member

1 2 3 4   Kept drinking when you promised yourself not to
1 2 3 4   Felt you were going crazy
1 2 3 4   Had a bad time

1 2 3 4   Felt physically or psychologically dependent on alcohol
1 2 3 4   Was told by a friend, neighbor or relative to stop or cut down drinking

Chapter 4

Impairment

Brief Impairment Scale (BIS)

Time 10 minutes

Ages 4–17

Time Frame Flexible, but not less than 3 months

Purpose Assessment of functional impairment.

Commentary

The BIS was designed to assess functional impairment, but instead linking impairment to specific disorders, the BIS is a global measure.

Versions

The Brief Impairment Scale (BIS) is intended to be administered to parents by an interviewer, but has the potential for self-adminstration.

Properties

Items The BIS comprises 23 items rated on a 4-point scale with responses for most items: no problem, some problem, a considerable problem, and a serious problem.

Scales The items of the BIS are scored on three subscales which are labeled: interpersonal relations, school/work, and self-fulfillment. In addition, all items can be scored on the total scale.

Reliability Test–retest intraclass correlations across a 12-day interval were 0.56 for the interpersonal relations subscale, 0.54 for the school/work subscale, 0.76 for the self-fulfillment subscale, and 0.70 for the total scale.

Cronbach's alphas ranged from 0.73 to 0.81 for the interpersonal relations subscale, from 0.76 to 0.81 for the school/work subscale, from 0.56 to 0.73 for the self-fulfillment subscale, and from 0.81 to 0.88 for the total scale.

Validity Correlations between the BIS total scale and a clinician-reported measure of impairment were significant and ranged from –0.52 to –0.53.

The BIS scores for mental health service users were significantly higher than the scores of nonservice users.

Norms

A table with cut-off values which discriminate between clinician-indicated impaired and nonimpaired children and between mental health service users and nonusers is given in Bird et al. (2005). These results are based on a single ethnic group. The authors recommend piloting the cut-off value in the population in which the instrument is to be used.

Use No supplemental materials available.

Key references

Bird HR, Canino GJ, Davies M, et al. The Brief Impairment Scale (BIS): A multidimensional scale of functional impairment for children and adolescents. J Am Acad Child Adolesc Psychiatry 2005; 44: 699–707.

Address

Hector R. Bird
New York State Psychiatric Institute (Unit 78)
1051 Riverside Drive
New York, NY 10032
USA
birdh@childpsych.columbia.edu

Brief Impairment Scale (BIS)

The questions I am going to ask you <u>now</u> have to do with how _____(name of child)_____ has been doing overall. Please answer them thinking <u>only</u> of the **last twelve months/past year** keeping in mind what one would expect of children of the same age and sex as _____(name of child)

1) **Over the last 12 months/year how much of a problem has he/she had getting along with his/her father/step-father/foster father? (score about father figure with whom he/she has most contact) (Read options):**
   0 no problem
   1 some problem
   2 a considerable problem
   3 a serious problem
   7 refused
   8 not applicable (no father figure)
   9 don't know

2) **How much of a problem has he/she had getting along with his/her mother/step-mother/foster mother? (score about mother figure with whom he/she has most contact) (Read options):**
   0 no problem
   1 some problem
   2 a considerable problem
   3 a serious problem
   7 refused
   8 not applicable (no mother figure)
   9 don't know

3) **How about problems getting along with his/her brothers and sisters?**
   0 no problem
   1 some problem
   2 a considerable problem
   3 a serious problem
   7 refused
   8 not applicable (no brothers or sisters)
   9 don't know

4) **How about getting involved in activities together with the rest of the family? (Read options):**
   0 no problem
   1 some problem
   2 a considerable problem
   3 a serious problem
   7 refused
   9 don't know

5) **Over the last 12 months/past year, how much of a problem has he/she had with his/her teachers at school? (If not in school and working) or with his/her superiors at work?**
   0 no problem
   1 some problem
   2 a considerable problem
   3 a serious problem
   7 refused
   8 not applicable (has not worked or been in school during the past year)
   9 don't know

6) **How much of a problem has he/she had getting along with other adults outside of the family? (Read options):**
   0 no problem
   1 some problem
   2 a considerable problem
   3 a serious problem
   7 refused
   9 don't know

7) **How much of a problem has he/she had making friends?**
   0 no problem
   1 some problem
   2 a considerable problem
   3 a serious problem
   7 refused
   9 don't know

8) **How much of a problem has he/she had getting along with the friends that he/she has? (Read options):**
   0 no problem
   1 some problem
   2 a considerable problem
   3 a serious problem
   7 refused
   9 don't know

9) **During the last 12 months/past year, has he/she often missed school/work? (Read options):**
   0 never misses school/work
   1 occasionally (once a month or less)
   2 many times (2–4 times a month)
   3 quite frequently (more than 5 times per month)
   7 refused
   8 not applicable, not in school and not working during the last 12 months
   9 don't know
   If Q. 9 coded 1, 2, or 3, ask
   9A) was this because he/she was really sick
   0, No; 1, Yes (If 'yes', recode q.9 as '0')

10) **During the last 12 months/past year, how well has he/she been doing in his/her school work? (Read options)**
    (If another grading system is used, code closest equivalent)
    0 better than average (mostly B's or outstanding: mostly A's, some B's
    1 just average: C work
    2 somewhat below average (mostly C's and D's)
    3 markedly below average (mostly D's and F's)
    7 refused
    8 not applicable (not in school during the past year)
    9 don't know
    If Q. 10 scored 8, ask 10A. Has he/she dropped out of school during the last year?
    0, no; 3, yes; 7, refused; 9, don't know
    (If 'Yes', code '3' for q.10)

11) **Has he/she been suspended from school during the last 12 months/past year?**
    0 no
    3 yes
    7 refused
    8 not applicable (has not been in school over the past year)
    9 don't know

12) **Has he/she been expelled from school or actually fired from a job during the last 12 months/past year?**
    0 no
    3 yes
    7 refused
    8 not applicable (has not been in school over the past year)
    9 don't know

13) **In general, how much of a problem has he/she had getting his/her schoolwork/work done on time? (Read options):**
  0 no problem
  1 some problem
  2 a considerable problem
  3 a serious problem
  7 refused
  8 not applicable (not in school or working over the past year)
  9 don't know

14) **During the last 12 months/past year, how much of a problem has he/she had doing what he/she is expected to do at home? (Read options):**
  0 no problem
  1 some problem
  2 a considerable problem
  3 a serious problem
  7 refused
  9 don't know

15) **How much of a problem has he/she had being responsible at school/work or in jobs he/she took on outside of his/her home? (Read options):**
  0 no problem
  1 some problem
  2 a marked problem
  3 a serious problem
  7 refused
  8 not applicable (not worked or in school during past year)
  9 don't know

16) **In the last 12 months/past year, how many times were you asked to come to his/her school to discuss some problem that he/she had?**
  0 never
  1 once
  3 more than once
  7 refused
  8 not applicable, not in school
  9 don't know

17) **To what extent does he/she get involved in sports? (Read options):**
  0 frequently or member of a team
  1 some involvement, but not steady
  2 very rarely involved
  3 not involved at all
  7 refused
  8 not applicable, no opportunities for participation in sports
  9 don't know

18) **Over the past 12 months/last year, to what extent did he/she get involved in activities other than sports? (Read options):**
  0 frequently involved in other activities
  1 only occasionally
  2 rarely got involved or dropped out easily
  3 never got involved in other activities
  7 refused
  9 don't know

19) **To what extent would you say he/she is a person who has many interests? Again think specifically about the last 12 months/past year. Would you say he/she (Read options):**
  0 has many and varied interests
  1 has some interests
  2 few things interest him/her
  3 has no interests, is generally bored
  7 refused
  9 don't know

20) **Compared to other kids of the same age, how neat is his/her physical appearance most of the time? Remember that we are talking of how it's been during the last 12 months/past year. Would you say he/she is (Read options):**
  0 like most kids his/her age
  1 a bit sloppier than most kids his/her age
  2 considerably more sloppy or peculiar than most
  3 extremely sloppy or bizarre compared to others
  7 refused
  9 don't know

21) **Compared to others his/her age, how well does he/she take care of his/her health? He/she (Read options):**
  0 takes good care of him/herself
  1 is somewhat careless about his/her health
  2 is quite careless about his/her health
  3 is extremely careless about his/her health
  7 refused
  9 don't know

22) **How safety conscious is he/she? (Read options):**
  0 very careful, attentive to safety rules
  1 somewhat careless
  2 quite careless
  3 extremely careless
  7 refused
  9 don't know

23) **Does he/she seem to have a problem having fun and enjoying life? Again, think of how it's been during the last 12 months/past year. Would you say he/she has had (Read options):**
  0 no problem
  1 some problem
  2 a considerable problem
  3 a serious problem
  7 refused
  9 don't know

Interpersonal Subscale: Items 1,2,3,4,5,6,7,8 School/work Subscale: Items 9,10,11,12,13,14,15,16 Self Subscale: Items 17,18,19,20,21,22,23

Scoring instructions
1) Each valid item must have been scored 0, 1, 2, or 3. Refusals (7), Not applicables (8), or Don't knows (9) are not summed in the score. (For the scale a subscale to be valid, at least half of the items have to have valid scores.)
2) For the total scale or for each subscale, add the sum of the valid items, divide by the number of valid items, and multiply times the number of items on the scale or subscale.

The scale is in the public domain.

Child and Adolescent Functional Assessment Scale (CAFAS)

Time 10 minutes

Ages 5–18

Time Frame Defined by user, typically last month or last three months

Purpose Assessment of impairment.

Commentary

The CAFAS was designed to assess children's functional impairment in several domains. Impairment is defined as the degree of interference of children's problems with their daily functioning. The CAFAS may be useful for designing treatment plans, conducting outcome studies, and evaluating service use. A downward extension of the CAFAS is also available: the Preschool and Early Childhood Functional assessment Scale (PECFAS) for ages 3–7 years.

Versions

The Child and Adolescent Functional Assessment Scale (CAFAS) is only available as a clinician report.

Properties

Items   The CAFAS comprises 8 subscales pertaining to children's functioning each consisting of 4 severity levels: severe, moderate, mild, and minimal or no impairment. Each subscale and severity level comprises a set of items describing behavior. A rater starts by reviewing items in the severe level of each subscale first and continues to lower levels until an item within a level describes a child's functioning. The level of that item indicates the impairment for that subscale. In addition to subscales for children's functioning, the CAFAS comprises 2 subscales pertaining to caregiver's functioning.

Scales   The subscales for children's functioning are: School/Work, Home, Community, Behavior Towards Others, Moods/Emotions, Self-Harmful Behavior, Substance Use, and Thinking. A total score consists of the sum of the 8 subscale scores. The subscales for caregiver's functioning are: Material Need, and Family/Social Support.

Reliability   Interrater correlations of ratings by students and clinicians with a criterion score ranged from 0.92 to 0.96 for the total score, and from 0.73 to 0.99 for the subscale scores. Correlation between ratings by different students on different occasions was 0.91 for the total score, and correlations ranged from 0.79 to 1.00 for the subscale scores.

Cronbach's alphas for the total score ranged from 0.63 to 0.78 in samples of clinical children.

Validity   Total scores of the CAFAS were significantly higher for inpatients than for children receiving home-based treatment, whose scores were in turn significantly higher than scores of outpatients. Children with more serious psychiatric disorders had significantly higher total scores than children with less serious psychiatric disorders.

Higher scores on the CAFAS were significantly associated with more restrictive care, higher cost, more bed days, and more days of services.

Norms   No information available.

Use   The CAFAS, an instructional manual, and a computer program for scoring and reporting are available from Kay Hodges at the address below.

Key references

Hodges K. Child and Adolescent Functional Assessment Scale (CAFAS) In: Maruish ME (ed.) The use of psychological testing for treatment planning and outcome assessment, 3rd edn. Mahwah, NJ: Lawrence Erlbaum Associates, 2004: 405–441.

Hodges K, Wong MM. Psychometric characteristics of a multidimensional measure to assess impairment: The Child and Adolescent Functional Assessment Scale. J Child Fam Stud 1996; 5: 445–67.

Address

Kay Hodges
Department of Psychology
Eastern Michigan University
2140 Old Earhart Road
Ann Arbor, MI 48105
USA
hodges@provide.net

Children's Global Assessment Scale (CGAS)

Time 1 minute

Ages 4–16

Time Frame Last month

Purpose Assessment of global functioning.

Commentary

The CGAS is an adaptation of the Global Assessment Scale (GAS) for adults developed by Endicott et al. (1976).

Versions

The Children's Global Assessment Scale (CGAS) was intended as a clinician's rating scale, but adaptations for interviewers and parents were used as well.

Properties

Items   The CGAS comprises one item that is rated on a 100-point scale. For each decile, the instrument contains behaviorally oriented descriptive examples.

Scales   The CGAS has no subscales. Raters assign one score ranging from 1 to 100.

Reliability   Test–retest intraclass correlations across a 6-month interval ranged from 0.69 to 0.95.

Interrater intraclass correlations across raters at two occasions were 0.84 and 0.85.

Validity   The CGAS correlated significantly with other clinician-rated measures of impairment and correlations

ranged from 0.76 to 0.92. Correlations between the CGAS and parent-reported measures of psychiatric problems were significant and were –0.65 and –0.62. The correlation between the CGAS and a parent-reported measure of hyperactivity was not significant.

The mean CGAS scores of inpatients were significantly lower, indicating worse functioning, than outpatients.

Norms   A cut-off value of 60 or lower on the CGAS is indicative of definite impairment.

Use   No supplemental materials available.

Key references

Bird HR, Canino G, Rubio-Stipec M. Ribera JC. Further measures of the psychometric properties of the Children's Global Assessment Scale. Arch Gen Psychiatry 1987; 44: 821–4.

Endicott J, Spitzer RL, Fleiss JL, Cohen J. The Global Asessment Scale: A procedure for measuring overall severity of psychiatric disturbance. Arch Gen Psychiatry 1976; 33: 766–71.

Shaffer D, Gould MS, Brasic J, et al. A Children's Global Assessment Scale (CGAS). Arch Gen Psychiatry 1983; 40: 1228–31.

Address

David Shaffer
New York State Psychiatric Institute (Unit 78)
1051 Riverside Drive
New York, NY 10032
USA
shafferd@childpsych.columbia.edu

Children's Global Assessment Scale (CGAS)

(for Children 4 to 16 Years of Age*)

Rate the subject's most impaired level of general functioning for the specified time period by selecting the *lowest* level which describes his/her functioning on a hypothetical continuum of health-Illness. Use Intermediary levels (eg, 35, 88, 62).

Rate actual functioning regardless of treatment or prognosis. The examples of behavior provided are only illustrative and are not required for a particular rating.

Specified Time Period: 1 mo

100–91 *Superior functioning* in all areas (at home, at school, and with peers); Involved in a wide range of activities and has many interests (eg, has hobbies or participates in extracurricular activities or belongs to an organized group such as Scouts, etc); likeable, confident; 'everyday' worries never get out of hand; doing well In school; no symptoms

90–81 *Good functioning* in all areas, secure in family, school, and with peers; there may be transient difficulties and 'everyday' worries that occasionally get out of hand (e.g., mild anxiety associated with an important exam, occasionally 'blowups' with siblings, parents, or peers)

80–71 *No more than slight impairment in functioning* at home, at school, or with peers; some disturbance of behavior or emotional distress may be present in response to life stresses (eg, parental separations, deaths, birth of a sib), but these are brief and interference with functioning is transient; such children are only minimally disturbing to others and are not considered deviant by those who know them

70–61 *Some difficulty in a single area*, but generally functioning pretty well (eg, sporadic or isolated antisocial acts, such as occasionally playing hooky or petty theft; consistent minor difficulties with school work; mood changes of brief duration; (ears and anxieties which do not lead to gross avoidance behavior; self-doubts); has some meaningful interpersonal relationships; most people who do not know the child well would not consider him/her deviant but those who do know him/her well might express concern

60–51 *Variable functioning with sporadic difficulties or symptoms in several but not all social areas*; disturbance would be apparent to those who encounter the child in a dysfunctional setting or time but not to those who see the child In other settings

50–41 *Moderate degree ol interference in functioning in most social areas or severe impairment of functioning in one area*, such as might result from, for example, suicidal preoccupations and ruminations, school refusal and other forms of anxiety, obsessive rituals, major conversion symptoms, frequent anxiety attacks, poor or inappropriate social skills, frequent episodes of aggressive or other antisocial behavior with some preservation of meaningful social relationships

40–31 *Major impairment in functioning in several areas and unable to function in one at these areas*, ie, disturbed at home, at school, with peers, or in society at large, e.g., persistent aggression without clear instigation; markedly withdrawn and isolated behavior due to either mood or thought disturbance, suicidal attempts with clear lethal intent; such children are likely to require special schooling and/or hospitalization or withdrawal from school (but this is not a sufficient criterion for inclusion in this category)

30–21 *Unable to function in almost all areas*, eg, stays at home, in ward, or in bed all day without taking part in social activities or severe impairment In reality testing or serious impairment in communication (eg, sometimes incoherent or inappropriate)

20–11 *Needs considerable supervision* to prevent hurting others or self (eg, frequently violent, repeated suicide attempts) or to maintain personal hygiene or gross impairment in all forms of communication, eg, severe abnormalities in verbal and gestural communication, marked social aloofness, stupor, etc

10–1 *Needs constant supervision* (24-hr care) due to severely aggressive or self-destructive behavior or gross impairment in reality testing, communication, cognition, affect, or personal hygiene

The scale is in the public domain.

Columbia Impairment Scale (CIS)

Time 5 minutes

Ages 4–16

Time Frame Flexible, but not less than 3 months

Purpose Assessment of functioning.

Commentary

The CIS was designed to assess multiple dimensions of functioning. While most measures of functioning rely on clinician's judgments, the CIS is a respondent-based measure.

Versions

The Columbia Impairmet Scale (CIS) comprises two forms: a form administered to parents and a self-report form administered to children or adolescents.

Properties

Items   The CIS comprises 13 items tapping four areas of functioning: interpersonal relations, psychopathology, functioning at school or work, and use of leisure time. The items are rated on a 5-point scale, but only three response labels are given: no problem, some problem, and a very big problem.

Scales   Factor analysis of the CIS items suggested one factor, so the items of the CIS are only scored on a total score.

Reliability   Test–retest intraclass correlations across 15–19-days intervals were 0.89 for the parent-report CIS, and 0.63 for the self-report CIS.

Cronbach's alphas on two occasions were 0.85 and 0.89 for the parent-report CIS, and 0.70 and 0.78 for the self-report CIS.

Validity   The parent-report CIS correlated moderately to high with other indicators of psychological dysfunction. The canonical correlation with the total set of indicators was 0.81. The correlations of the indicators with the self-report CIS were lower than with the parent-report CIS. The canonical correlation was 0.51.

The mean scores of the CIS differed significantly between clinical subjects and community subjects on two occasions. The difference was greater for the parent-report CIS than for the self-report CIS. ROC analysis showed a strong correspondence between the parent-report CIS and a clinician's rating of impairment.

Norms   A cut-off value of 15 or greater on the CIS is indicative of definite impairment.

Use   No supplemental materials available.

Key references

Bird HR, Shaffer D, Fisher P, et al. The Columbia Impairment Scale (CIS): Pilot findings on a measure of global impairment for children and adolescents. Int J Methods Psychiatr Res 1993; 3: 167–76.

Address

Hector R. Bird
New York State Psychiatric Institute (Unit 78)
1051 Riverside Drive
New York, NY 10032
USA
birdh@childpsych.columbia.edu

Columbia Impairment Scale (CIS)

In general, how much of a problem do you think [he/she] has with:

1.	getting into trouble	0	I	2	3	4	
2.	getting along with you ([his/her]) mother?	0	I	2	3	4	8
3.	getting along with [his/her] father (you)?	0	I	2	3	4	8
4.	feeling unhappy or sad?	0	I	2	3	4	

How much of a problem would you say he/she has:

5.	with his/her behavior at school (or job)?	0	I	2	3	4	8
6.	with having fun?	0	I	2	3	4	
7.	getting along with adults other than you or his/her father/mother?	0	I	2	3	4	

How much of a problem does he/she have:

8.	with feeling nervous or worried?	0	I	2	3	4	
9.	getting along with his/her brother(s)/sister(s)?	0	I	2	3	4	8
10.	getting along with other kids his/her age?	0	I	2	3	4	

How much of a problem would you say he/she has:

11.	getting involved in activities like sports or hobbies?	0	I	2	3	4	
12.	with his/her schoolwork (doing his/her job)?	0	I	2	3	4	8
13.	with his/her behavior at home?	0	I	2	3	4	

Response options provided: 0, no problem; 1–3, some problem; 4, a very big problem; 8 (not applicable).
The scale is in the public domain.

Functional Impairment Scale for Children and Adolescents (FISCA)

Time 30–40 minutes

Ages 5–18

Time Frame Not specified

Purpose Assessment of impairment.

Commentary

The FISCA is modeled on the Child and Adolescent Functional Assessment Scale (CAFAS; Hodges, 2004), but was modified into a parent and self-report to eliminate interviewer and rater involvement.

Versions

The Functional Impairment Scale for Children and Adolescents (FISCA) is available as a parent report and self-report (FISCA-SR).

Properties

Items   The FISCA and FISCA-SR comprise 183 items of which most are rated on a yes-no scale or a 3-point scale with responses: never, occasionally, and often.

Scales   The items are scored on 8 subscales: School, Home, Delinquency, Thinking, Control of Aggression, Feelings & Moods, Self-Harm, and Alcohol & Drugs. A total score, Total Impairment, is computed by summing all subscale scores. Factor analysis was used to determine the structure of the 8 subscales. The analysis indicated that the subscales could be combined into 3 composite scales: Undercontrolled Aggression, Social Role Violations, and Self-focused Impairment.

Reliability   Test–retest correlations across a 3-month interval ranged from 0.16 to 0.75 for parent-reported subscales and the correlation was 0.45 for Total Impairment in a sample of clinical children.

Cronbach's alphas ranged from 0.54 to 0.87 for parent-reported subscales, except the Home subscale (0.28), and the alpha was 0.50 for Total Impairment in a sample of clinical children. Alphas ranged from 0.61 to 0.88 for self-reported subscales, except the Home subscale (0.26).

Validity   Absolute values of correlations of the composite scales ranged for Undercontrolled Aggression from 0.15 to 0.23 with corresponding clinician-rated scales and from 0.07 to 0.14 with noncorresponding scales, ranged for Social Role Violations from 0.18 to 0.21 with corresponding scales and from 0.03 to 0.16 with noncorresponding scales, and ranged for Self-focused Impairment from 0.09 to 0.14 with corresponding scales and from 0.01 to 0.10 with noncorresponding scales.

The FISCA significantly predicted hospital recidivism, i.e. discharged patients returning to the hospital within a certain time.

Norms   No information available.

Use   The FISCA can be obtained from Susan J. Franks at the address below.

Key references

Franks SJ, Paul JS, Marks M, Van Egeren LA. Initial validation of the Functional Impairment Scale for Children and Adolescents. J Am Acad Child Adolesc Psychiatry 2000; 39: 1300–8.

Frank SJ, Van Egeren LA, Fortier JL, Chase P. Structural, relative, and absolute agreement between parents' and adolescent inpatients' reports of adolescent functional impairment. J Abnorm Child Psychol 2000; 28: 395–402.

Hodges K. Child and Adolescent Functional Assessment Scale (CAFAS) In: Maruish ME (ed.) The use of psychological testing for treatment planning and outcome assessment, 3rd edn. Mahwah, NJ: Lawrence Erlbaum Associates, 2004: 405–41.

Van Egeren LA, Frank SJ, Paul JS. Daily ratings among child and adolescent inpatients: The Abbreviated Child Behavior Rating Form. J Am Acad Child Adolesc Psychiatry 1999; 38: 1414–25.

Address

Susan J. Frank
Department of Psychology
Michigan State University
East Lansing, MI 48824
USA
franks@msu.edu

Health of the Nation Outcome Scales for Children and Adolescents (HoNOSCA)

Time 5 minutes

Ages 3–18

Time Frame Last 2 weeks

Purpose Assessment of impairment.

Commentary

The HoNOSCA was designed as a brief instrument to assess health and social functioning to be used in routine clinical practice by mental health practitioners.

Versions

The Health of the Nation Outcome Scales for Children and Adolescents (HoNOSCA) are available as a clinician report, a parent-report, and a self-report.

Properties

Items The HoNOSCA comprises two sections. The first section comprises 13 items about problems and impairment, and the optional second section comprises 2 items covering lack of information about difficulties and services. The second section is omitted from the parent report and self-report. The items of the clinician report are rated on a 5-point scale with responses: no problem, minor problem requiring no action, mild problem but definitely present, moderately severe problem, and severe to very severe problem. There is a glossary available that explains response options for clinicians. The items of the parent report and self report are rated on a 5-point scale with response: not at all, insignificantly, mild but definitely, moderately, and severely.

Scales The items of the first section are scored on 4 subscales which are supported by factor analysis. The subscales are: Behavior, Impairment, Symptoms, and Social. In addition to the subscales, a total score can be computed by summing the 13 item ratings.

Reliability Test–retest correlations across a 1-week interval ranged from 0.32 to 0.88 for the self-reported items and the correlation was 0.81 for the total score among adolescent inpatients.

Interrater intraclass correlations among three raters ranged from 0.67 to 0.98 for clinician-rated items.

Split-half reliability was 0.73 for the self-reported total score among adolescent inpatients.

Validity The clinician-reported total score correlated 0.60 with another clinician-rated measure of impairment. The self-reported total score correlated 0.66 with self-reported emotional and behavioural problems.

Inpatients' scores were significantly higher than outpatients' scores. Inpatients' clinician-reported and self-reported total scores were significantly lower at discharge than at admission to hospital.

Norms No information available.

Use Rating scales and the glossary for clinicians can be downloaded from the website at the address below. The website provides extensive information about the HoNOSCA as well.

Key references

Gowers S, Bailey-Rogers SJ, Shore A, Levine W. The Health of the Nation Outcome Scales for Child & Adolescent mental health (HoNOSCA). Child Psychol Psychiat Rev 2000; 5: 50–6.

Gowers S, Harringtom RC, Whitton A, et al. Brief scale for measuring the ourcomes of emotional and behavioural disorders in children: Health of the Nation Outcome Scales for Children and Adolescents (HoNOSCA). Br J Psychiatry 1999; 174: 413–16.

Gowers S, Levine W, Bailey-Rogers SJ, Shore A, Burhouse E. Use of a routine, self-report outcome measure (HoNOSCA-SR) in two adolescent mental health services. Br J Psychiatry 2002; 180: 266–9.

Address

Simon Gowers
Academic Unit
Pine Lodge
79 Liverpool Road
Chester CH2 1AW
UK
sgowers@liv.ac.uk
www.liv.ac.uk/honosca

Which scale to use and when

Assessment scales	Abbreviation	Informants	Number of items	Administration time (minutes)
General rating scales				
Achenbach System of Empirically Based Assessment	ASEBA	Parent, teacher, self	100–120	10–20
Behavioral Assessment System for Children – Second Edition	BASC-2	Parent, teacher, self	100–185	10–30
Brief Psychiatric Rating Scale for Children	BPRS-C	Clinician	21	5
Child Symptom Inventories	CSI	Parent, teacher, self	79–120	15–20
Conners' Rating Scales – Revised	CRS-R	Parent, teacher, self	Long: 59–87 Short: 27–28	15–20
Devereux Scales of Mental Disorders	DSMD	Parent, teacher	110–111	20
Pediatric Symptom Checklist	PSC	Parent, self	35	5
Revised Behavior Problem Checklist	RBPC	Parent, teacher	89	15
Strengths and Difficulties Questionnaire	SDQ	Parent, teacher, self	25	5
Anxiety problems				
Affect and Arousal Scale	AFARS	Self	27	5
Childhood Anxiety Sensitivity Index	CASI	Self	18	5
Fear Survey Schedule for Children – Revised	FSSR-C	Self	80	15
Kutcher Generalized Social Anxiety Disorder Scale for Adolescents	K-GSADS-A	Clinician	32	15
Liebowitz Social Anxiety Scale for Children and Adolescents	LSAS-CA	Clinician	24	10
Multidimensional Anxiety Scale for Children	MASC	Self	Standard: 39 Short: 10	15
Pediatric Anxiety Rating Scale	PARS	Clinician	57	30
Penn State Worry Questionnaire for Children	PSWQ-C	Self	14	5
Physical Arousal Scale for Children and Positive and Negative Affect Scale for Children	PH-C, PANAS-C	Self	45	15
Revised Child Anxiety and Depression Scale	RCADS	Self	47	10
Revised Children's Manifest Anxiety Scale	RCMAS	Self	37	5–10
Screen for Child Anxiety Related Emotional Disorders	SCARED	Parent, self	41	10
Social Anxiety Scale for Children – Revised, Social Anxiety Scale for Adolescents	SASC-R, SAS-A	Parent, self	22	10
Social Phobia and Anxiety Inventory for Children	SPAI-C	Self	63	20–30
Spence Children's Anxiety Scale	SCAS	Parent, self	45	5–10
State-Trait Anxiety Inventory for Children	STAIC	Self	40	20
Obsessive Compulsive Disorders				
Children's Obsessional Compulsive Inventory	CHOCI	Self	30	15
Children's Yale–Brown Obsessive Compulsive Scale	CY-BOCS	Clinician	10	5
Leyton Obsessional Inventory – Child Version	LOI-CV	Self	Standard: 44, Survey: 20, Short: 11	10
Depression				
Children's Depression Inventory	CDI	Self, parent, teacher	Original: 27, short: 10, extensions: 12–17	5–10
Children's Depression Rating Scale – Revised	CDRS-R	Clinician	17	10
Children's Depression Scale	CDS	Self, parent, teacher, clinician	Self, parent: 50; teacher, clinician: 10	5–40
Depression Self-Rating Scale	DSRS	Self	18	5
Kutcher Adolescent Depression Scale	KADS	Self	6–16	5
Mood and Feelings Questionnaire	MFQ	Parent, self	Standard: 32 Short: 13	3–10
Reynolds Child Depression Scale, Reynolds Adolescent Depression Scale – 2nd Edition	RCDS, RADS-2	Self	30	5–10

Ages	Time frame *	Purpose	Rating scale reproduced **	Page
1½–18	Last 6 months	Assessment of competence, adaptive functioning, emotional and behavioral problems	Full scale	17
2–21	NS	Assessment of emotional and behavioral problems, adaptive functioning and personality	No	23
5–18	NS	Assessment of emotional and behavioral problems	Journal	25
3–18	NS	Assessment of emotional and behavioral problems	Sample items	26
3–17	Last month	Assessment of emotional and behavioral problems	Sample items	29
5–18	Last 4 weeks	Assessment of emotional and behavioral problems	No	31
4–16	NS	Assessment of emotional and behavioral problems	Full scale	32
5–18	NS	Assessment of emotional and behavioral problems	Sample items	35
4–16	Last 6 months	Assessment of emotional and behavioral problems	Website	36
7–18	NS	Assessment of positive and negative affect and physiological arousal	Full scale	39
8–15	NS	Assessment of belief that anxiety symptoms have negative consequences	Full scale	41
8–16	NS	Assessment of phobic fears	Full scale	43
11–17	NS	Assessment of social anxiety problems	Full scale	46
7–18	NS	Assessment of social anxiety and avoidance	No	48
8–19	NS	Assessment of anxiety problems	Sample items	49
6–17	Last week	Assessment of the severity of anxiety symptoms	Full scale	51
6–18	NS	Assessment of worry	Full scale	55
10–18	Last 2 weeks, last few weeks	Assessment of positive and negative affect and physiological arousal	Full scale	57
6–18	NS	Assessment of anxiety and depression symptoms corresponding to dimensions of several DSM-IV anxiety disorders and major depression	Full scale	59
6–19	NS	Assessment of anxiety problems	Sample items	61
9–18	Last 3 months	Assessment of anxiety symptoms	Full scale	62
6–18	NS	Assessment of social anxiety problems	No	65
8–14	NS	Assessment of social anxiety problems	Sample items	67
7–19	NS	Assessment of anxiety symptoms consistent with DSM-IV classification	Website	69
Grades 4–6	State=now, trait=usually	Assessment of state and trait anxiety	Sample items	70
7–17	NS	Assessment of obsessive and compulsive problems	Journal	71
4–18	Last week	Assessment of severity of obsessive and compulsive symptoms	Full scale	76
13–18	NS	Assessment of obsessive and compulsive symptoms	Full scale	80
7–17	Last 2 weeks	Assessment of depressive problems	Sample items	82
6–12	NS	Assessment of depressive symptoms	Sample items	84
7–18	NS	Assessment of depressive problems	No	86
8–14	Last week	Assessment of depressive symptoms	Full scale	87
12–20	Last week	Assessment of depressive problems	Full scale	89
8–18	Last 2 weeks	Assessment of depressive problems	Website	92
8–20	Last 2 weeks	Assessment of depressive problems	Sample items	93

Assessment scales	Abbreviation	Informants	Number of items	Administration time (minutes)
Suicide				
Child-Adolescent Suicidal Potential Index	CASPI	Self	30	10
Multi-Attitude Suicide Tendency Scale	MAST	Self	30	10
Positive and Negative Suicide Ideation Inventory	PANSI	Self	14	5
Suicidal Behaviors Questionnaire-Revised	SBQ-R	Self	5	5
Suicidal Ideation Questionnaire	SIQ	Self	15–30	5–10
Eating disorders				
Anorectic Behavior Observation Scale	ABOS	Parent	30	5
Children's Eating Attitude Test	ChEAT	Self	26	5
Children's Eating Behavior Inventory	CEBI	Parent	40	15
Children's Eating Behaviour Questionnaire	CEBQ	Parent	35	10
Questionnaire of Eating and Weight Patterns	QEWP	Parent, self	12	5
Tics				
Motor tic, Obsessions and compulsions, Vocal tic Evaluation Survey	MOVES	Self	20	5
Tourette's Disorder Scale	(TODS)	Parent, clinician	15	15
Yale Global Tic Severity Scale	YGTSS	Clinician	10	10
Developmental disorders				
Asperger Syndrome Diagnostic Scale	ASDS	Parent, teacher	50	10–15
Autism Behavior Checklist	ABC	Parent, teacher	57	10
Autism Spectrum Screening Questionnaire	ASSQ	Parent, teacher	27	10
Behavioral Summarized Evaluation – Revised	BSE-R	Raters	29	5–10
Checklist for Autism in Toddlers	CHAT	Parent, clinician	14	15
Childhood Asperger Syndrome Test	CAST	Parent	44	10–15
Childhood Autism Rating Scale	CARS	Parent, clinician	15	5
Children's Communication Checklist-Second Edition	CCC-2	Parent	70	5–15
Gilliam Asperger's Disorder Scale	GADS	Parent, professional	52	10
Gilliam Autism Rating Scale – Second Edition	GARS-2	Parent, professional	62	10
Infant Behavioral Summarized Evaluation	IBSE	Clinician	33	10–15
Krug Asperger's Disorder Index	KADI	Parent, professional	32	5
Modified Checklist for Autism in Toddlers	M-CHAT	Parent	23	5
PDD Behavior Inventory	PDDBI	Parent, teacher	Standard: 120–124 Extended: 180–188	20–45
Pervasive Developmental Disorders Screening Test-II	PDDST-II	Parent	12–22	15
Real Life Rating Scale	RLRS	Raters	47	10–15
Social Communication Questionnaire	SCQ	Parent	40	10
Social Responsiveness Scale	SRS	Parent, teacher	65	15
ADHD				
ADHD Rating Scale-IV	ADHD RS-IV	Parent, teacher	18	5
ADHD Symptoms Rating Scale	ADHD-SRS	Parent, teacher	56	10–15
Attention Deficit Disorders Evaluation Scale – Third Edition	ADDES-3	Parent, teacher	46–60	20
Attention-Deficit/Hyperactivity Disorder Test	ADHDT	Parent, teacher, professional	36	5–10
Brown Attention-Deficit Disorder Scales	Brown ADD Scales	Parent, teacher, self	40–50	10–20
IOWA Conners Teacher's Rating Scale	IOWA Conners	Teacher	10	5
Swanson, Kotkin, Atkins, M-Flynn, and Pelham	SKAMP	Teacher, observer	10	5
Swanson, Nolan, and Pelham-IV	SNAP-IV	Parent, teacher	90	15
Vanderbilt ADHD Diagnostic Parent Rating Scales, Vanderbilt ADHD Diagnostic Teacher Rating Scales	VADPRS, VADTRS	Parent, teacher	35–47	10

Ages	Time frame *	Purpose	Rating scale reproduced **	Page
6–18	Last 6 months	Assessment of risks for suicidal behavior	No	95
14–24	NS	Assessment of suicidal behavior	Full scale	96
14–19	Last 2 weeks	Assessment of positive and negative thoughts related to suicide	Website	98
14–17	Lifetime, last year, future	Assessment of suicidal behaviors	Website	100
Grades 7–12	Last month	Assessment of suicidal ideation	Sample items	101
14–24	Last month	Assessment of eating behaviors and attitudes	Full scale	102
Grades 3–8	NS	Assessment of eating behavior	Full scale	104
2–12	NS	Assessment of eating behavior	Full scale	106
3–18	NS	Assessment of eating style	Full scale	108
12–18	Last 6 months	Assessment of eating behavior	Journal	110
7–20	Last week	Assessment of tics	Journal	113
6–17	Last week	Assessment of tics and comorbid symptoms	Full scale	114
5–51	Last week	Assessment of tics	Full scale	116
5–18	NS	Assessment of behaviors associated with Asperger syndrome	Sample items	119
1_-35	NS	Assessment of autistic behaviors	Sample items	120
6–17	NS	Assessment of autistic behaviors	Full scale	121
1½-12	Last 5 days	Assessment of autistic behavior	No	123
18 months	NS	Assessment of autistic behavior	Full scale	127
4–11	NS	Assessment of behaviors associated with Asperger syndrome	Full scale	129
0–18	NS	Assessment of autistic behaviors	Sample items	131
4–16	Last week	Assessment of communication problems	No	133
3–22	NS	Assessment of Asperger's disorder behavior	Sample items	135
3–22	NS	Assessment of autistic behaviors	Sample items	137
½-4	NS	Assessment of autistic behaviors	Journal	139
6–21	NS	Assessment of Asperger's disorder behavior	Sample items	140
18–30 months	NS	Assessment of autistic behaviors	Journal	141
1½-12½	NS	Assessment of problem behaviors and social communication skills	Sample items	143
1½-8	Birth–36 months	Assessment of autistic behaviors	No	145
6–16	30–minutes periods	Assessment of autistic behaviors	Full scale	146
4–40	Last 3 months, lifetime	Assessment of autistic behaviors	Sample items	148
4–18	Last 6 months	Assessment of autistic behaviors	Sample items	150
4–20	Last 6 months	Assessment of ADHD problems	No	152
5–18	Last 3 months	Assessment of ADHD problems	Sample items	154
4–18	NS	Assessment of ADHD problems	Sample items	156
3–23	NS	Assessment of ADHD problems	Sample items	158
3–18	Last 6 months	Assessment of ADHD problems	Sample items	160
Grades K–6	NS	Assessment of disruptive problems	Full scale	162
6–12	Current	Assessment of ADHD problems	Website	164
6–12	NS	Assessment of ADHD problems	Website	165
6–12	NS	Assessment of disruptive problems	Full scale	166

Assessment scales	Abbreviation	Informants	Number of items	Administration time (minutes)
Conduct disorder				
Antisocial Process Screening Device	APSD	Parent, teacher	20	10
Children's Aggression Scales	CAS	Parent, teacher	23–33	10
Children's Social Behavior Scale	CSBS	Peer, teacher	13–15	10
Direct and Indirect Aggression Scale	DIAS	Self, peer	24	5
Eyberg Child Behavior Inventory, Sutter–Eyberg Student Behavior Inventory-Revised	ECBI, SESBI-R	Parent, teacher	36–38	10
Home Situations Questionnaire, School Situations Questionnaire	HSQ, SSQ	Parent, teacher	12–16	5
New York Rating Scales	NYRS	Parent, teacher	36–47	15
Proactive and Reactive Aggression Scale	PRAS	Teacher	6	1
Substance Use				
Adolescent Alcohol and Drug Involvement Scale	AADIS	Self	30	10
Adolescent Substance Abuse Subtle Screening Inventory – Second Version	SASSI-A2	Self	100	15
Personal Experience Inventory	PEI	Self	300	45–55
Personal Experience Screening Questionnaire	PESQ	Self	40	10
Rutgers Alcohol Problem Index	RAPI	Self	18, 23	10
Impairment				
Brief Impairment Scale	BIS	Parents	23	10
Child and Adolescent Functional Assessment Scale	CAFAS	Clinician	8	10
Children's Global Assessment Scale	CGAS	Clinician	1	1
Columbia Impairmet Scale	CIS	Parent, self	13	5
Functional Impairment Scale for Children and Adolescents	FISCA	Parent, self	183	30–40
Health of the Nation Outcome Scales for Children and Adolescents	HoNOSCA	Clinician, parent, self	13–15	5

* NS = Not Specified
** Full scale = Full scale reprinted here
Website = Full scale can be found on website
Journal = Full scale reprinted in referenced journal paper
Sample items = Sample items reprinted here
No = Not available

Ages	Time frame *	Purpose	Rating scale reproduced **	Page
6–13	NS	Assessment of psychopathy problems	Sample items	170
6–12	Last year	Assessment of aggressive behaviors	Full scale	172
9–12	NS	Assessment of social aggression	No	176
8–15	NS	Assessment of social aggression	Website	177
2–16	Current	Assessment of disruptive problems	Sample items	178
4–11	NS	Assessment of disruptive problems	No	180
3–17	Last 4 weeks	Assessment of disruptive behavior and positive peer relations	Sample items	181
Grades 1–6	NS	Assessment of aggressive behavior	Full scale	183
11–17	NS	Assessment of alcohol and drug involvement	Full scale	185
12–18	Last 6, months, lifetime, specific periods	Assessment of substance use problems	Full scale	188
12–18	NS	Assessment of drug involvement, accompanying psychosocial problems, and drug history	Sample items	192
12–18	NS	Assessment of drug involvement, accompanying psychosocial problems, and drug history	Sample items	195
12–21	Last year, can be varied	Assessment of problem drinking	Full scale	197
4–17	Flexible	Assessment of functional impairment	Full scale	201
5–18	Optional	Assessment of impairment	No	204
4–16	Last month	Assessment of global functioning	Full scale	205
4–16	Flexible	Assessment of functioning	Full scale	207
5–18	NS	Assessment of impairment	No	209
3–18	Last 2 weeks	Assessment of impairment	Website	210

Appendix 2

Alphabetic list of scales